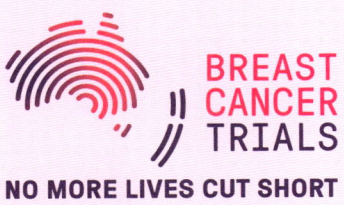

NO MORE LIVES CUT SHORT

The Australian Women's Health Diary
funds breast cancer clinical trials research
to save and improve the lives of
every person affected by breast cancer.

Today, tomorrow and forever.

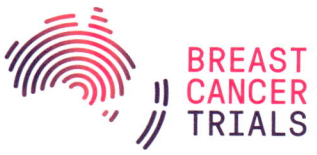

Imagine a world without breast cancer… Now imagine that in your lifetime

A breast cancer diagnosis is devastating. It doesn't matter how old you are; no one expects to have their life put at risk.

Everyone wants and deserves their future.

In Australia, nine women still lose their life to breast cancer every day, leaving heartbroken families and friends behind.

Every one of them matters.

It is the most commonly diagnosed cancer in the world – every minute of every day, another person is being told they have breast cancer.

Breast cancer is cruel. It is complicated and we don't have all the answers.

We need more solutions for every person, every situation, every time.

Clinical trials research is the proven pathway to get new breast cancer treatments to patients and those at risk.

We have a bold ambition for a future where no one dies from breast cancer.

Where no more lives are cut short.

It's going to take time, passion, new ways of thinking, inspiration, determination and a community behind us, but we won't give up until no more lives are cut short.

Thank you for buying this diary and for working with us to achieve this. We wish you a safe, healthy and happy year ahead.

THE TEAM AT BREAST CANCER TRIALS

FIND OUT MORE AT BREASTCANCERTRIALS.ORG.AU OR SCAN THIS CODE

Calendar 2026

JANUARY
S	M	T	W	T	F	S
				1	2	3
4	5	6	7	8	9	10
11	12	13	14	15	16	17
18	19	20	21	22	23	24
25	26	27	28	29	30	31

FEBRUARY
S	M	T	W	T	F	S
1	2	3	4	5	6	7
8	9	10	11	12	13	14
15	16	17	18	19	20	21
22	23	24	25	26	27	28

MARCH
S	M	T	W	T	F	S
1	2	3	4	5	6	7
8	9	10	11	12	13	14
15	16	17	18	19	20	21
22	23	24	25	26	27	28
29	30	31				

APRIL
S	M	T	W	T	F	S
			1	2	3	4
5	6	7	8	9	10	11
12	13	14	15	16	17	18
19	20	21	22	23	24	25
26	27	28	29	30		

MAY
S	M	T	W	T	F	S
31					1	2
3	4	5	6	7	8	9
10	11	12	13	14	15	16
17	18	19	20	21	22	23
24	25	26	27	28	29	30

JUNE
S	M	T	W	T	F	S
	1	2	3	4	5	6
7	8	9	10	11	12	13
14	15	16	17	18	19	20
21	22	23	24	25	26	27
28	29	30				

JULY
S	M	T	W	T	F	S
			1	2	3	4
5	6	7	8	9	10	11
12	13	14	15	16	17	18
19	20	21	22	23	24	25
26	27	28	29	30	31	

AUGUST
S	M	T	W	T	F	S
30	31					1
2	3	4	5	6	7	8
9	10	11	12	13	14	15
16	17	18	19	20	21	22
23	24	25	26	27	28	29

SEPTEMBER
S	M	T	W	T	F	S
		1	2	3	4	5
6	7	8	9	10	11	12
13	14	15	16	17	18	19
20	21	22	23	24	25	26
27	28	29	30			

OCTOBER
S	M	T	W	T	F	S
				1	2	3
4	5	6	7	8	9	10
11	12	13	14	15	16	17
18	19	20	21	22	23	24
25	26	27	28	29	30	31

NOVEMBER
S	M	T	W	T	F	S
1	2	3	4	5	6	7
8	9	10	11	12	13	14
15	16	17	18	19	20	21
22	23	24	25	26	27	28
29	30					

DECEMBER
S	M	T	W	T	F	S
		1	2	3	4	5
6	7	8	9	10	11	12
13	14	15	16	17	18	19
20	21	22	23	24	25	26
27	28	29	30	31		

My goals and hopes for this year

What would you like to achieve in 2026? Write down your goals and how you plan to accomplish them, making changes or additions throughout the year as needed.

MY GOALS AND HOPES	TO ACHIEVE THEM I NEED TO...

2025

JANUARY
S	M	T	W	T	F	S
			1	2	3	4
5	6	7	8	9	10	11
12	13	14	15	16	17	18
19	20	21	22	23	24	25
26	27	28	29	30	31	

FEBRUARY
S	M	T	W	T	F	S
						1
2	3	4	5	6	7	8
9	10	11	12	13	14	15
16	17	18	19	20	21	22
23	24	25	26	27	28	

MARCH
S	M	T	W	T	F	S
30	31					1
2	3	4	5	6	7	8
9	10	11	12	13	14	15
16	17	18	19	20	21	22
23	24	25	26	27	28	29

APRIL
S	M	T	W	T	F	S
		1	2	3	4	5
6	7	8	9	10	11	12
13	14	15	16	17	18	19
20	21	22	23	24	25	26
27	28	29	30			

MAY
S	M	T	W	T	F	S
				1	2	3
4	5	6	7	8	9	10
11	12	13	14	15	16	17
18	19	20	21	22	23	24
25	26	27	28	29	30	31

JUNE
S	M	T	W	T	F	S
1	2	3	4	5	6	7
8	9	10	11	12	13	14
15	16	17	18	19	20	21
22	23	24	25	26	27	28
29	30					

JULY
S	M	T	W	T	F	S
		1	2	3	4	5
6	7	8	9	10	11	12
13	14	15	16	17	18	19
20	21	22	23	24	25	26
27	28	29	30	31		

AUGUST
S	M	T	W	T	F	S
31					1	2
3	4	5	6	7	8	9
10	11	12	13	14	15	16
17	18	19	20	21	22	23
24	25	26	27	28	29	30

SEPTEMBER
S	M	T	W	T	F	S
	1	2	3	4	5	6
7	8	9	10	11	12	13
14	15	16	17	18	19	20
21	22	23	24	25	26	27
28	29	30				

OCTOBER
S	M	T	W	T	F	S
			1	2	3	4
5	6	7	8	9	10	11
12	13	14	15	16	17	18
19	20	21	22	23	24	25
26	27	28	29	30	31	

NOVEMBER
S	M	T	W	T	F	S
30						1
2	3	4	5	6	7	8
9	10	11	12	13	14	15
16	17	18	19	20	21	22
23	24	25	26	27	28	29

DECEMBER
S	M	T	W	T	F	S
	1	2	3	4	5	6
7	8	9	10	11	12	13
14	15	16	17	18	19	20
21	22	23	24	25	26	27
28	29	30	31			

2027

JANUARY
S	M	T	W	T	F	S
31					1	2
3	4	5	6	7	8	9
10	11	12	13	14	15	16
17	18	19	20	21	22	23
24	25	26	27	28	29	30

FEBRUARY
S	M	T	W	T	F	S
	1	2	3	4	5	6
7	8	9	10	11	12	13
14	15	16	17	18	19	20
21	22	23	24	25	26	27
28						

MARCH
S	M	T	W	T	F	S
	1	2	3	4	5	6
7	8	9	10	11	12	13
14	15	16	17	18	19	20
21	22	23	24	25	26	27
28	29	30	31			

APRIL
S	M	T	W	T	F	S
				1	2	3
4	5	6	7	8	9	10
11	12	13	14	15	16	17
18	19	20	21	22	23	24
25	26	27	28	29	30	

MAY
S	M	T	W	T	F	S
30	31					1
2	3	4	5	6	7	8
9	10	11	12	13	14	15
16	17	18	19	20	21	22
23	24	25	26	27	28	29

JUNE
S	M	T	W	T	F	S
		1	2	3	4	5
6	7	8	9	10	11	12
13	14	15	16	17	18	19
20	21	22	23	24	25	26
27	28	29	30			

JULY
S	M	T	W	T	F	S
				1	2	3
4	5	6	7	8	9	10
11	12	13	14	15	16	17
18	19	20	21	22	23	24
25	26	27	28	29	30	31

AUGUST
S	M	T	W	T	F	S
1	2	3	4	5	6	7
8	9	10	11	12	13	14
15	16	17	18	19	20	21
22	23	24	25	26	27	28
29	30	31				

SEPTEMBER
S	M	T	W	T	F	S
			1	2	3	4
5	6	7	8	9	10	11
12	13	14	15	16	17	18
19	20	21	22	23	24	25
26	27	28	29	30		

OCTOBER
S	M	T	W	T	F	S
31					1	2
3	4	5	6	7	8	9
10	11	12	13	14	15	16
17	18	19	20	21	22	23
24	25	26	27	28	29	30

NOVEMBER
S	M	T	W	T	F	S
	1	2	3	4	5	6
7	8	9	10	11	12	13
14	15	16	17	18	19	20
21	22	23	24	25	26	27
28	29	30				

DECEMBER
S	M	T	W	T	F	S
			1	2	3	4
5	6	7	8	9	10	11
12	13	14	15	16	17	18
19	20	21	22	23	24	25
26	27	28	29	30	31	

Personal information

IF FOUND PLEASE CONTACT:

NAME

ADDRESS

STATE　　POSTCODE

PHONE NUMBER　　MOBILE

EMAIL

IN CASE OF EMERGENCY:

NAME

TELEPHONE　　MOBILE

USEFUL TELEPHONE NUMBERS:

DOCTOR	GAS
DENTIST	ELECTRICITY
VET	WATER
CHILD CARE	PLUMBER
SCHOOL	MECHANIC

OTHER IMPORTANT INFORMATION:

Key contacts

NAME
ADDRESS
STATE   POSTCODE
TELEPHONE (H)   (W)
MOBILE   EMAIL

NAME
ADDRESS
STATE   POSTCODE
TELEPHONE (H)   (W)
MOBILE   EMAIL

NAME
ADDRESS
STATE   POSTCODE
TELEPHONE (H)   (W)
MOBILE   EMAIL

NAME
ADDRESS
STATE   POSTCODE
TELEPHONE (H)   (W)
MOBILE   EMAIL

NAME
ADDRESS
STATE   POSTCODE
TELEPHONE (H)   (W)
MOBILE   EMAIL

NAME
ADDRESS
STATE   POSTCODE
TELEPHONE (H)   (W)
MOBILE   EMAIL

Key contacts

NAME

ADDRESS

STATE POSTCODE

TELEPHONE (H) (W)

MOBILE EMAIL

NAME

ADDRESS

STATE POSTCODE

TELEPHONE (H) (W)

MOBILE EMAIL

NAME

ADDRESS

STATE POSTCODE

TELEPHONE (H) (W)

MOBILE EMAIL

NAME

ADDRESS

STATE POSTCODE

TELEPHONE (H) (W)

MOBILE EMAIL

NAME

ADDRESS

STATE POSTCODE

TELEPHONE (H) (W)

MOBILE EMAIL

NAME

ADDRESS

STATE POSTCODE

TELEPHONE (H) (W)

MOBILE EMAIL

Special events 2026

JANUARY

FEBRUARY

MARCH

APRIL

MAY

JUNE

JULY

AUGUST

SEPTEMBER

OCTOBER

NOVEMBER

DECEMBER

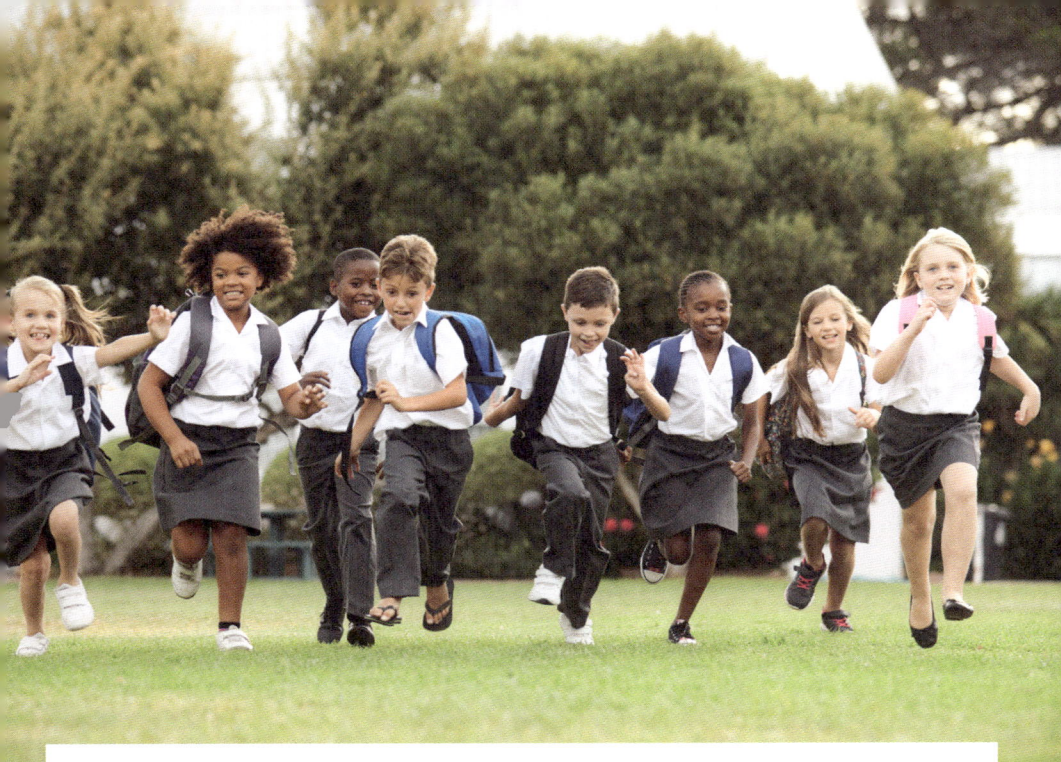

School terms 2026

NEW SOUTH WALES

- **TERM 1** January 27 – April 2
- **TERM 2** April 20 – July 3
- **TERM 3** July 20 – September 25
- **TERM 4** October 12 – December 17

AUSTRALIAN CAPITAL TERRITORY

- **TERM 1** January 29 – April 2
- **TERM 2** April 20 – July 3
- **TERM 3** July 20 – September 25
- **TERM 4** October 12 – December 18

QUEENSLAND

- **TERM 1** January 22 – April 2
- **TERM 2** April 16 – June 26
- **TERM 3** July 13 – September 18
- **TERM 4** October 6 – December 11

VICTORIA

- **TERM 1** January 27 – April 2
- **TERM 2** April 20 – June 26
- **TERM 3** July 13 – September 18
- **TERM 4** October 5 – December 18

WESTERN AUSTRALIA

- **TERM 1** February 2 – April 2
- **TERM 2** April 20 – July 3
- **TERM 3** July 20 – September 25
- **TERM 4** October 12 – December 17

NORTHERN TERRITORY

- **TERM 1** January 27 – April 2
- **TERM 2** April 13 – June 19
- **TERM 3** July 13 – September 18
- **TERM 4** October 5 – December 11

SOUTH AUSTRALIA

- **TERM 1** January 27 – April 10
- **TERM 2** April 27 – July 3
- **TERM 3** July 20 – September 25
- **TERM 4** October 12 – December 11

TASMANIA

- **TERM 1** February 2 – April 17
- **TERM 2** May 4 – July 10
- **TERM 3** July 27 – October 2
- **TERM 4** October 19 – December 21

CHECK WITH YOUR SCHOOL FOR DATES OF PUPIL-FREE DAYS

Budget planner 2026

$$$	WEEKLY	MONTHLY	ANNUALLY
INCOME			
Net salary/wage			
Bonuses (after tax)			
Dividends/income from investments			
Interest			
Other			
TOTAL INCOME			
EXPENDITURE			
HOUSEHOLD			
Rent/mortgage			
Council rates			
Water rates			
Power & heating			
Telephone & internet			
House & contents insurance			
Maintenance/repairs			
Other			
PERSONAL			
Groceries			
Clothing			
Child care			
School fees			
Toiletries/cosmetics/haircare/massage			
Newspapers/magazines			
Superannuation			
Other			
LOANS			
Personal loans			
Credit/after pay			
Other			

$$$	WEEKLY	MONTHLY	ANNUALLY
TRANSPORT			
Public transport			
Car registration			
Car insurance			
Petrol			
Tolls			
Parking			
Other			
HEALTH			
Doctor/dentist/other specialists			
Health insurance			
Chemist			
Life insurance/income protection			
Other			
ENTERTAINMENT			
Eating out			
Concerts/movies/theatre			
Memberships			
Holidays			
Hobbies			
Streaming services			
Other			
OTHER			
Gifts			
Donations to charity			
Regular investments			
Savings/rainy day fund			
TOTAL EXPENDITURE			
TOTAL INCOME			
INCOME MINUS EXPENDITURE			

DATE OF MY NEXT BUDGET REVIEW   /   /

Health checklist

	LOOKING FOR	**HOW OFTEN**
Eye examination	Vision loss, general eye health and conditions like glaucoma and cataracts.	Every 2-3 years from age 40 and yearly from age 65. More regularly if there is a family history of glaucoma, diabetes or high blood pressure.
Dental	Gum disease, cavities and general decline in dental health.	Every 6-12 months for a check-up and clean, or more often for gum issues or plaque build-up.
Hearing	Hearing loss.	When you notice hearing damage or have concerns, or annually for those aged 60 and over.
Bone density scan	Osteoporosis or low bone density.	Consult your GP if you are aged over 50 and have a high risk of osteoporosis.
Immunisation	Immunity to influenza, Covid-19, tetanus, rubella, shingles etc.	As advised by your GP. Flu shots are available yearly, and are free for those aged over 65.
Cervical Screening Test	Signs of the human papillomavirus (HPV) and cervical cancer.	From age 25-74 if you are or have ever been sexually active. If results are normal, continue to be tested every five years thereafter.
STI test	Common sexually transmitted diseases, such as chlamydia, gonorrhoea, syphilis, genital herpes, hepatitis B and HIV.	Every six to 12 months if you're sexually active, have a new partner, frequently change partners, travel to areas with a high prevalence of STIs or have been exposed in the last 12 months.
Breast self-examination	Breast changes, lumps, dimpling or thickening of the skin, nipple change or discharge, pain.	Know the normal look and feel of your breasts. If you notice any new or unusual changes, see your GP, particularly if they persist.
Screening mammogram	Breast lumps or changes not evident to the touch.	Every two years from age 50-74, or annually and earlier if at high risk of breast cancer.
Diabetes screening	Elevated blood glucose levels.	Screening is dependent on your individual risk level. Ask your GP for advice.
Skin check	Spots, moles and freckles which are dry, scaly or have smudgy borders.	Self-check on a regular basis and see your GP about any new or changed skin lesions. Get checked opportunistically if you work outdoors.
Bowel cancer screening	Polyps, other signs of bowel cancer.	Faecal occult blood test every two years from age 50-74, plus a five-yearly colonoscopy. Early testing is available for those deemed to be at moderate risk of bowel cancer; ask your GP.
Blood pressure	High blood pressure, which can increase risk of heart disease and stroke; low blood pressure.	Every two years for healthy adults aged 18 and over, or more often if there's a family history of high blood pressure, stroke, kidney or heart disease.
Cholesterol	High LDL (bad cholesterol) and triglycerides, and low HDL (good cholesterol).	Every five years from age 45, or every 12 months if you're at risk of cardiovascular disease. The results, along with your BP results, will be interpreted by your GP in the context of your overall absolute cardiovascular risk.
Body Mass Index	Healthy weight range and waist measurement.	Every two years by your GP or more often if part of an identified or increased risk group.

LAST CHECKED	CONTACT	DATE OF APPOINTMENT	COMPLETED
	For more information, visit health.gov.au/ncsp or call 1800 627 701		
	BreastScreen Australia: 132 050		
	For more information, visit health.gov.au/nbcsp or call 1800 627 701		

Aboriginal and Torres Strait Islander people may have different health needs; discuss these with your doctor.

Don't forget

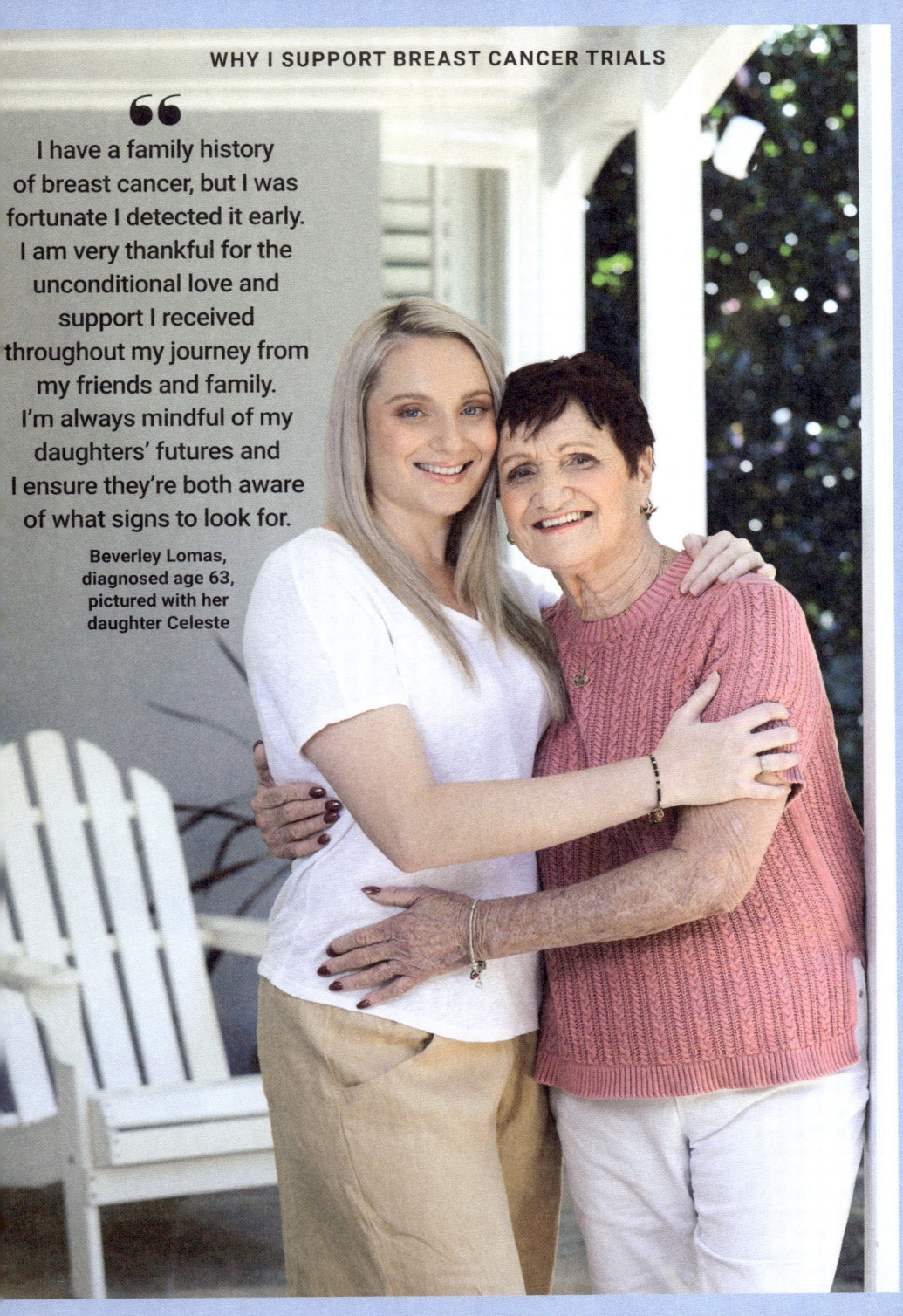

WHY I SUPPORT BREAST CANCER TRIALS

> I have a family history of breast cancer, but I was fortunate I detected it early. I am very thankful for the unconditional love and support I received throughout my journey from my friends and family. I'm always mindful of my daughters' futures and I ensure they're both aware of what signs to look for.

Beverley Lomas, diagnosed age 63, pictured with her daughter Celeste

let's talk about HEALTHY HABITS

As a new year begins, it's a good time to set some goals that prioritise your health and happiness. Be flexible and remember, the best resolutions are the ones that suit your interests and lifestyle.

When life gets busy or motivation wanes, these practical steps could help you stay on track.

1 PLAN FOR EXERCISE

Doing some form of exercise each day will do wonders for your mind and body, and plotting your workouts into your diary can help ensure they don't get forgotten. Think creatively to find windows in your schedule, whether it means setting your alarm an hour early, going to the gym in your lunch break or combining social catch-ups with a walk.

2 MAKE WATER EASILY ACCESSIBLE

It's easy to neglect your water intake when you're busy with other things, so try leaving glasses and carafes within reach. Keep a glass of water by your bed or desk, have water jugs chilling in the fridge and carry a bottle with you when out and about.

3 MEAL PLAN AND PREP

Having a fridge and pantry stocked with healthy options will limit the temptation to snack on sugary treats or order takeaway. Use the weekend to plan out your meals, shop for ingredients and prepare what you can ahead of time. Wash fresh produce and store in airtight containers, pre-chop vegetables, cook some meals ready for the week or whip up a batch of healthy muffins.

4 PRIORITISE SLEEP

It's important to give your body time to rest and reboot each night so it's ready to tackle those health goals in the morning. Create a bedtime routine that includes a wind-down ritual like meditation, a cup of herbal tea or gentle stretches. Go to bed and wake up at the same time each day, allowing for your recommended seven to nine hours of sleep each night, and switch off screens two hours before bed.

BE KIND TO YOURSELF
Occasionally, life might throw a curveball in the form of illness, a family emergency or an unexpected errand or work crisis to derail your good intentions. Try not to let one bad day or missed opportunity get you down or destroy your momentum. Focus on the small wins and adapt your goals to the circumstances, reminding yourself that tomorrow is a new day and another opportunity to tick off what you may have missed out on today.

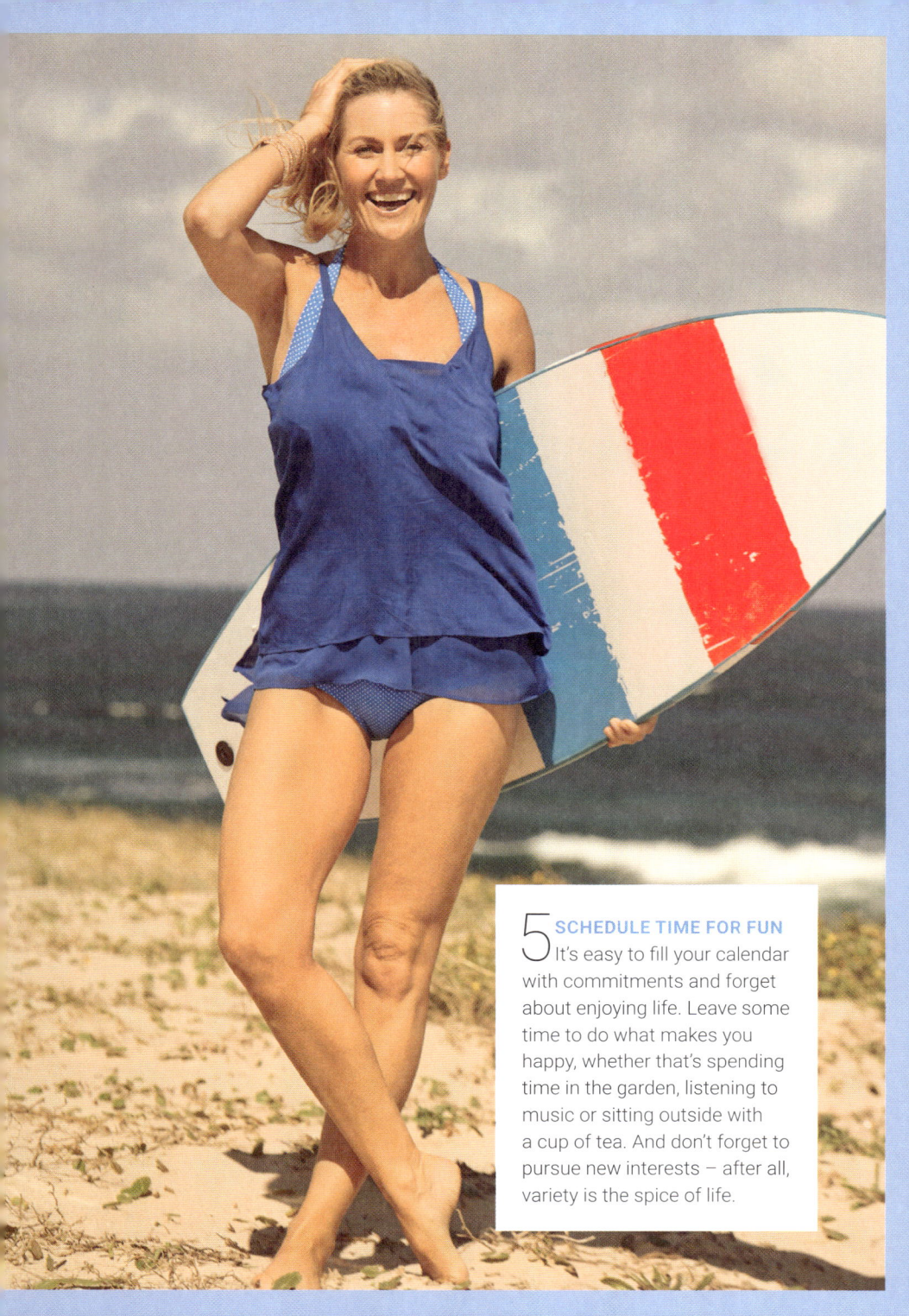

5 SCHEDULE TIME FOR FUN

It's easy to fill your calendar with commitments and forget about enjoying life. Leave some time to do what makes you happy, whether that's spending time in the garden, listening to music or sitting outside with a cup of tea. And don't forget to pursue new interests – after all, variety is the spice of life.

	DECEMBER					
S	M	T	W	T	F	S
	1	2	3	4	5	6
7	8	9	10	11	12	13
14	15	16	17	18	19	20
21	22	23	24	25	26	27
28	29	30	31			

	JANUARY					
S	M	T	W	T	F	S
				1	2	3
4	5	6	7	8	9	10
11	12	13	14	15	16	17
18	19	20	21	22	23	24
25	26	27	28	29	30	31

	FEBRUARY					
S	M	T	W	T	F	S
1	2	3	4	5	6	7
8	9	10	11	12	13	14
15	16	17	18	19	20	21
22	23	24	25	26	27	28

29 MONDAY

30 TUESDAY

31 WEDNESDAY NEW YEAR'S EVE

1 THURSDAY NEW YEAR'S DAY

January 2026

2 FRIDAY

3 SATURDAY

> **THANK YOU FOR PURCHASING THIS DIARY.**
> You're making our vital breast cancer research possible. Visit breastcancertrials.org.au/VIPDiaryOffer to receive your special gift.

4 SUNDAY

	DECEMBER					
S	M	T	W	T	F	S
	1	2	3	4	5	6
7	8	9	10	11	12	13
14	15	16	17	18	19	20
21	22	23	24	25	26	27
28	29	30	31			

	JANUARY					
S	M	T	W	T	F	S
				1	2	3
4	5	6	7	8	9	10
11	12	13	14	15	16	17
18	19	20	21	22	23	24
25	26	27	28	29	30	31

	FEBRUARY					
S	M	T	W	T	F	S
1	2	3	4	5	6	7
8	9	10	11	12	13	14
15	16	17	18	19	20	21
22	23	24	25	26	27	28

5 MONDAY

6 TUESDAY

7 WEDNESDAY

8 THURSDAY

January 2026

9 FRIDAY

10 SATURDAY

> **FORGET THE UNSUSTAINABLE NEW YEAR'S RESOLUTIONS** and set small goals instead. For example, eat more vegies, try a home workout or start a gratitude journal.

11 SUNDAY

		DEC	EMB	ER		
S	M	T	W	T	F	S
	1	2	3	4	5	6
7	8	9	10	11	12	13
14	15	16	17	18	19	20
21	22	23	24	25	26	27
28	29	30	31			

		JAN	UAR	Y		
S	M	T	W	T	F	S
				1	2	3
4	5	6	7	8	9	10
11	12	13	14	15	16	17
18	19	20	21	22	23	24
25	26	27	28	29	30	31

		FEB	RUA	RY		
S	M	T	W	T	F	S
1	2	3	4	5	6	7
8	9	10	11	12	13	14
15	16	17	18	19	20	21
22	23	24	25	26	27	28

12 MONDAY

13 TUESDAY

14 WEDNESDAY

15 THURSDAY

January 2026

16 FRIDAY ISRA AND MI'RAJ (ISLAMIC HOLY DAY)

17 SATURDAY

> **INVEST IN A FITNESS TRACKER** this year to help keep track of your step count, heart rate, water consumption, sleep patterns and more.

18 SUNDAY

	DECEMBER					
S	M	T	W	T	F	S
	1	2	3	4	5	6
7	8	9	10	11	12	13
14	15	16	17	18	19	20
21	22	23	24	25	26	27
28	29	30	31			

	JANUARY					
S	M	T	W	T	F	S
				1	2	3
4	5	6	7	8	9	10
11	12	13	14	15	16	17
18	19	20	21	22	23	24
25	26	27	28	29	30	31

	FEBRUARY					
S	M	T	W	T	F	S
1	2	3	4	5	6	7
8	9	10	11	12	13	14
15	16	17	18	19	20	21
22	23	24	25	26	27	28

19 MONDAY

20 TUESDAY

21 WEDNESDAY

22 THURSDAY

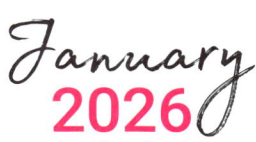
January 2026

23 FRIDAY

24 SATURDAY

AVOID THE TEMPTATION to check your phone as soon as you wake up. Leave it for at least an hour to start your day free of distractions.

25 SUNDAY

	D	E	C	E	M	B	E	R	
S	M	T	W	T	F	S
	1	2	3	4	5	6
7	8	9	10	11	12	13
14	15	16	17	18	19	20
21	22	23	24	25	26	27
28	29	30	31			

	J	A	N	U	A	R	Y
S	M	T	W	T	F	S
				1	2	3
4	5	6	7	8	9	10
11	12	13	14	15	16	17
18	19	20	21	22	23	24
25	26	27	28	29	30	31

	F	E	B	R	U	A	R	Y
S	M	T	W	T	F	S
1	2	3	4	5	6	7
8	9	10	11	12	13	14
15	16	17	18	19	20	21
22	23	24	25	26	27	28

26 MONDAY   AUSTRALIA DAY

27 TUESDAY

28 WEDNESDAY

29 THURSDAY

January – February 2026

30 FRIDAY

31 SATURDAY

> **EMBRACE ANCIENT SUPERFOODS** to boost energy, improve sleep and give your skin a healthy glow. Try fermented vegetables, bone broth or turmeric.

1 SUNDAY

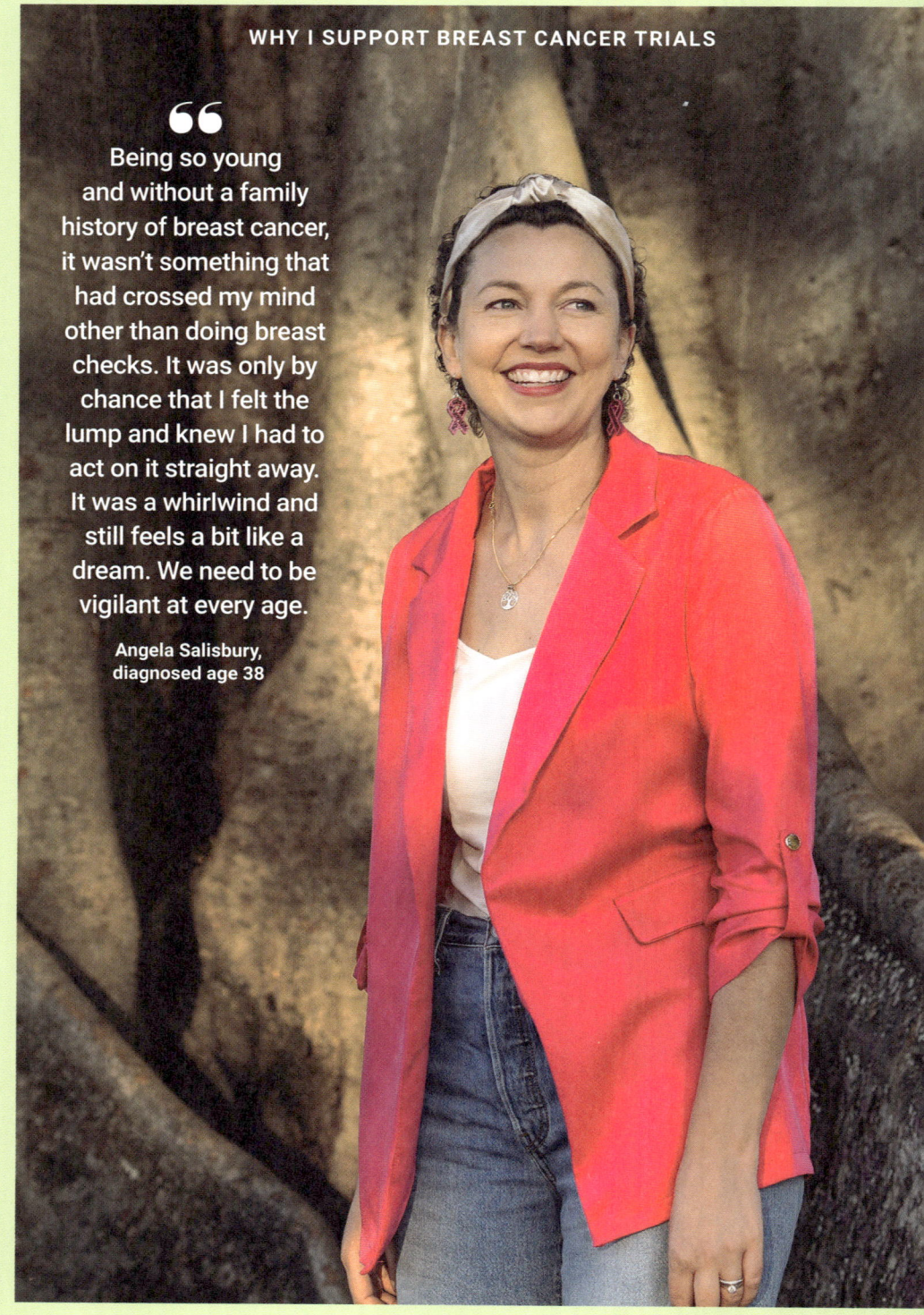

WHY I SUPPORT BREAST CANCER TRIALS

> Being so young and without a family history of breast cancer, it wasn't something that had crossed my mind other than doing breast checks. It was only by chance that I felt the lump and knew I had to act on it straight away. It was a whirlwind and still feels a bit like a dream. We need to be vigilant at every age.

Angela Salisbury, diagnosed age 38

let's talk about BEING ACTIVE

The benefits of getting regular exercise are many, including improving mental health, strengthening the heart, assisting with weight loss and boosting immune function. Enjoy the perks every day.

The recommended physical activity guidelines are as follows: to be active on most (if not all) days of the week and enjoy a total of 2.5 to 5 hours of moderate activity or 1.25 to 2.5 hours of vigorous activity per week, or a combination of both. Try these ideas to make those goals easier to achieve.

9 FUN WAYS TO MOVE MORE

1 **Walk and talk.** Whether you're taking a work call or phoning a friend, parent or child, take your chats on the go, rather than sitting idle. Watch for cars!

2 **Make it a social occasion.** Incorporate movement into social catch-ups. Think strolling around an art gallery, going for a bush walk or doing a yoga class together.

3 **Plan active dates.** Shake up your usual dinner and a movie routine with some active date-night options. Try dance lessons, walks along the beach, a game of tennis or orienteering.

4 **Make it a challenge.** Sign up for a fun run, charity walk or a triathlon to give yourself something to work towards while also raising money for a worthwhile cause.

5 **Try an after-dinner walk.** Change your couch-potato tendencies by heading out for a walk at the end of the day. Go alone for some me-time or take your kids or partner to catch up on the day's events.

6 **Hit the shops.** Run errands and add to your daily movement tally with a trip to the shops. Stick to local stores so you can walk there and back or park your car at the furthest point of the car park.

7 **Indulge your inner child.** Rediscover the unashamed delights of your youth. Dance to your favourite song, jump on the trampoline or play hopscotch.

8 **Make it a team effort.** You're more likely to exercise when you have others relying on you. Join a hiking club, sign up for a new sport or try geocaching.

9 **Take it outdoors.** Many outdoor chores like weeding, raking, mowing or washing the car count towards your exercise goals and they're great for your mental health, too. Play some tunes or listen to a podcast while you work.

For more information, visit Exercise Right; exerciseright.com.au

Exercise options for every age

It's recommended we enjoy 30 minutes of moderate-intensity physical activity every day, regardless of our age. But as our bodies and physical abilities change, so should our exercise choices. Consider the following options and check with an exercise professional if unsure.

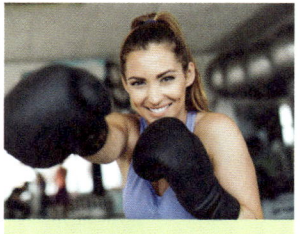

IN YOUR 20S
You may have greater freedom and time to dedicate to fitness. Aim for a variety of cardio and strength training for improved physical outcomes later in life.
TRY: Team sports, rowing, boxing, boot camp or a triathlon.

IN YOUR 30S
Muscle tone and mass may decline and posture can suffer if you have a desk job. Prioritise strength training twice a week as well as regular pelvic floor exercises.
TRY: High intensity interval training (HIIT), squats, lunges or yoga.

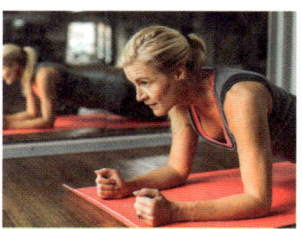

IN YOUR 40S
You might have less time to exercise and weight creep and back pain could become an issue. Focus on resistance exercises to burn calories and build muscle and core strength.
TRY: Running, weight training, stand-up paddle boarding or Pilates.

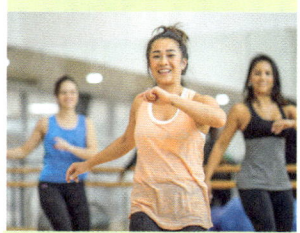

IN YOUR 50S
You'll enter menopause and be at greater risk of developing type 2 diabetes and cardiovascular disease. Incorporate strength training twice a week to maintain muscle and bone mass.
TRY: Walking, Zumba, cycling or tennis.

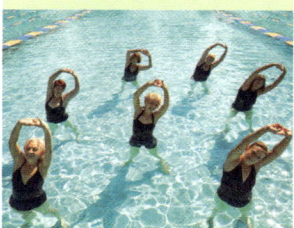

IN YOUR 60S
With chronic conditions more common and our cancer risk increasing, physical activity remains important. Prioritise exercises that build strength and flexibility.
TRY: Aquarobics, golf, resistance band exercises or gardening.

70S AND BEYOND
Exercise remains beneficial to help prevent falls, maintain cognitive function and keep you mobile. Seek advice from your healthcare provider as to the best kind for you.
TRY: Walking, water exercises, Tai Chi or an exercise physiology class.

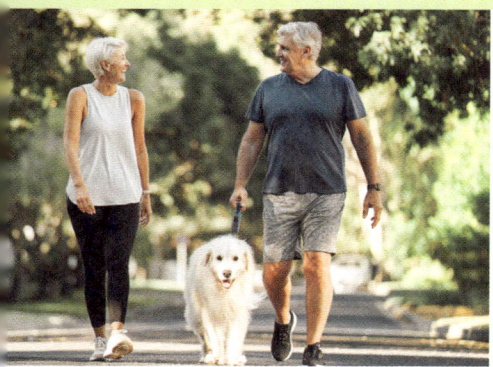
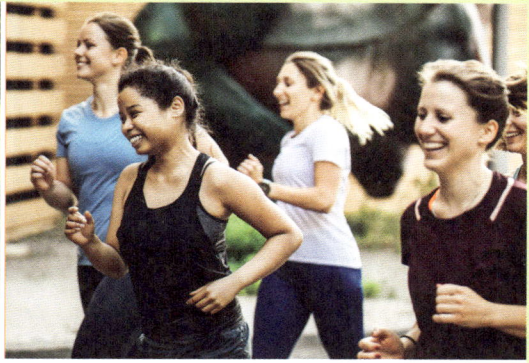

Walking vs running – which is better?

Whether you like to walk at a brisk pace or prefer to speed things up with a light jog, walking and running are both excellent forms of cardiovascular exercise. Read on to discover the advantages and advice for each option, and consider giving both a try.

WALKING	RUNNING
Classed as a moderate-intensity, low-impact form of physical activity.	Classed as a vigorous, high-impact form of physical activity.
Helps you burn kilojoules, however you need to walk at a brisk pace and for longer to gain the same fitness benefits as running.	Burns around double the kilojoules of walking, helping you to achieve your weight-loss goals faster.
You can walk almost anywhere as well as incidentally, such as walking to the bus or taking the stairs instead of the lift.	A great option if you're short on time and want an efficient exercise option. Run indoors on a treadmill or head outdoors.
Walking at a steady pace can boost cardiovascular health, extend your life span and reduce the risk of chronic disease.	Running can strengthen muscles, improve cardiovascular fitness, increase metabolism and help maintain a healthy weight.
It helps to lubricate and strengthen the muscles that support the joints, which is beneficial for those with arthritis or joint pain.	Due to it being a weight-bearing exercise, running can help protect the bones from osteoporosis later in life.
Many walkers report that walking outdoors gives them more time to think and inspires their creativity.	Running releases brain chemicals called endocannabinoids, which leave you in a relaxed state of bliss known as 'runner's high'.
Consider joining a walking group, signing up for a charity walk or doing guided walks of cities, gardens or national parks.	You may like to participate in fun runs, park runs or marathons. Contact your local running club to meet fellow runners.
If you walk for too long or beyond your capability, you may end up with shin splints or plantar fasciitis (heel inflammation).	Over time, overuse injuries can include stress fractures, ITB friction syndrome (runner's knee) or plantar fasciitis.
A good choice if you're new to exercise, walking is accessible for nearly all fitness levels and ages.	Check with your doctor if you're over 40, are overweight, have a chronic illness or past injury or haven't exercised in a long time.

Best exercises for bone health

Approximately 1.2 million people in Australia live with osteoporosis, and 6.3 million have low bone density. Exercise can help maintain bone health and reduce the risk of fractures, with weight-bearing exercises, resistance training and balance exercises most beneficial. Try these exercises, giving yourself at least a day between bouts to recover. Consult a personal trainer or exercise professional for the correct technique and to avoid injury.

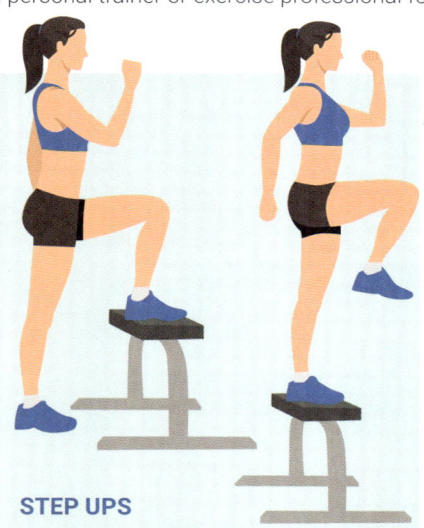

STEP UPS

Using a sturdy stool or step, place one foot on the step. Keep your back straight and push through the foot to lift your body onto the step. Step back to the start position and repeat on both legs.

SQUATS

Stand with feet slightly wider than shoulder-width apart, toes pointed out slightly and hands clasped in front. Slowly descend as if there is a chair behind you, bending at the hips, knees and ankles. Go as deep as you can, keeping knees in line with toes. Return to the starting position and repeat.

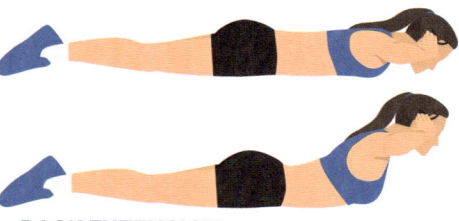

BACK EXTENSION

Lie on your stomach on a yoga mat or rug. Place your fingertips at your temples with elbows bent. Slowly raise your chest and arms, with your hips, legs and feet anchored to the floor; avoid straining your neck. Hold for five seconds then lower to start position. Repeat.

LUNGES

Stand with feet hip-width apart, engaging your core to maintain posture. Step forward with one leg, bend both knees and lower hips to the ground to create a 90-degree angle (or as close as you can). Push through the front foot to return to start position. Repeat on both legs. Add hand weights if able.

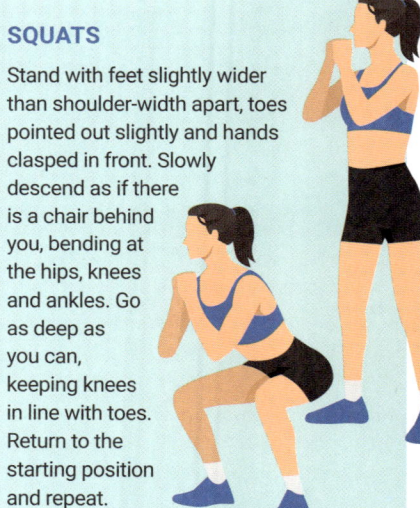

WE NEED YOUR FEEDBACK

Help us to keep in touch with what matters to you and ensure your diary remains relevant, practical and informative by completing our short online survey today.

You can also unlock special offers like pre-ordering your 2027 Australian Women's Health Diary at a discounted price!

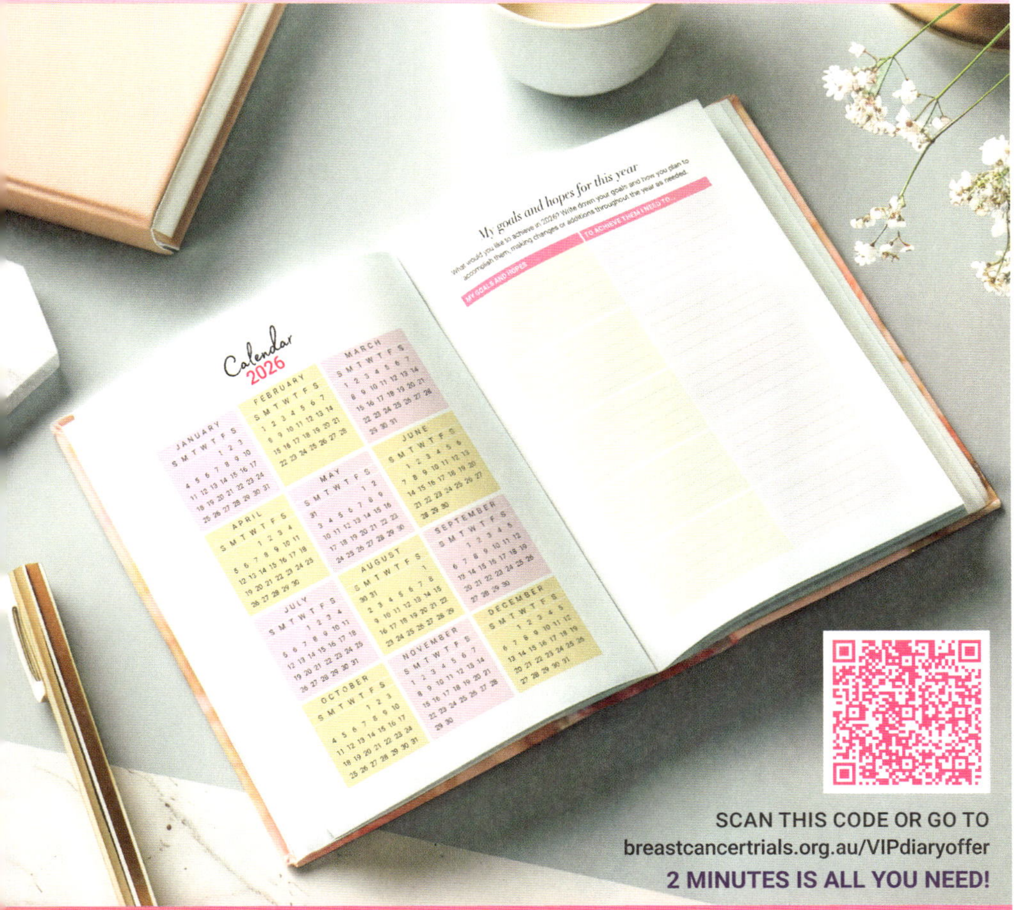

SCAN THIS CODE OR GO TO
breastcancertrials.org.au/VIPdiaryoffer
2 MINUTES IS ALL YOU NEED!

The Australian Women's Health Diary is an initiative of Breast Cancer Trials produced in conjunction with our friends at The Australian Women's Weekly. For 28 years, not only has this diary helped Australian women to be organised and informed about their health, it has also saved lives from breast cancer.

Learn more at breastcancertrials.org.au or call 1800 423 444.

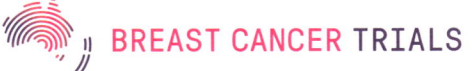

	JANUARY					
S	M	T	W	T	F	S
				1	2	3
4	5	6	7	8	9	10
11	12	13	14	15	16	17
18	19	20	21	22	23	24
25	26	27	28	29	30	31

	FEBRUARY					
S	M	T	W	T	F	S
1	2	3	4	5	6	7
8	9	10	11	12	13	14
15	16	17	18	19	20	21
22	23	24	25	26	27	28

	MARCH					
S	M	T	W	T	F	S
1	2	3	4	5	6	7
8	9	10	11	12	13	14
15	16	17	18	19	20	21
22	23	24	25	26	27	28
29	30	31				

2 MONDAY

3 TUESDAY

4 WEDNESDAY

5 THURSDAY

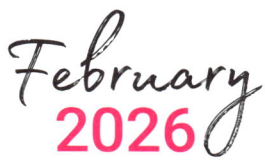

February 2026

6 FRIDAY

7 SATURDAY

> **NEW TO EXERCISE?** Start slowly and gradually progress the intensity as you feel ready. Do this by increasing the pace or distance or adding weights or resistance bands.

8 SUNDAY

	JANUARY					
S	M	T	W	T	F	S
				1	2	3
4	5	6	7	8	9	10
11	12	13	14	15	16	17
18	19	20	21	22	23	24
25	26	27	28	29	30	31

	FEBRUARY					
S	M	T	W	T	F	S
1	2	3	4	5	6	7
8	9	10	11	12	13	14
15	16	17	18	19	20	21
22	23	24	25	26	27	28

	MARCH					
S	M	T	W	T	F	S
1	2	3	4	5	6	7
8	9	10	11	12	13	14
15	16	17	18	19	20	21
22	23	24	25	26	27	28
29	30	31				

9 MONDAY ROYAL HOBART REGATTA (TAS)

10 TUESDAY

11 WEDNESDAY

12 THURSDAY

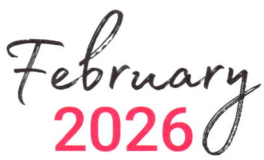

February 2026

13 FRIDAY

14 SATURDAY VALENTINE'S DAY

> **CHOOSE ACTIVE TOYS FOR YOUR CHILDREN** over sedentary activities. Think balls, frisbees, scooters, hula hoops, roller skates or skipping ropes.

15 SUNDAY

JANUARY						
S	M	T	W	T	F	S
				1	2	3
4	5	6	7	8	9	10
11	12	13	14	15	16	17
18	19	20	21	22	23	24
25	26	27	28	29	30	31

FEBRUARY						
S	M	T	W	T	F	S
1	2	3	4	5	6	7
8	9	10	11	12	13	14
15	16	17	18	19	20	21
22	23	24	25	26	27	28

MARCH						
S	M	T	W	T	F	S
1	2	3	4	5	6	7
8	9	10	11	12	13	14
15	16	17	18	19	20	21
22	23	24	25	26	27	28
29	30	31				

16 MONDAY

17 TUESDAY LUNAR NEW YEAR

18 WEDNESDAY RAMADAN BEGINS, LENT BEGINS

19 THURSDAY

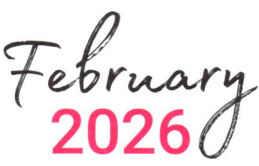

20 FRIDAY

21 SATURDAY

EXERCISE DOESN'T HAVE TO BE EXPENSIVE. Try free community classes or online workouts, explore outdoor gyms, swim in the ocean or go for a walk.

22 SUNDAY

	JANUARY					
S	M	T	W	T	F	S
				1	2	3
4	5	6	7	8	9	10
11	12	13	14	15	16	17
18	19	20	21	22	23	24
25	26	27	28	29	30	31

	FEBRUARY					
S	M	T	W	T	F	S
1	2	3	4	5	6	7
8	9	10	11	12	13	14
15	16	17	18	19	20	21
22	23	24	25	26	27	28

	MARCH					
S	M	T	W	T	F	S
1	2	3	4	5	6	7
8	9	10	11	12	13	14
15	16	17	18	19	20	21
22	23	24	25	26	27	28
29	30	31				

23 MONDAY

24 TUESDAY

25 WEDNESDAY

26 THURSDAY

February – March 2026

27 FRIDAY

28 SATURDAY

> **STAY SAFE.** Wear bright, reflective clothing if you're exercising on the street or footpaths at night, and avoid exercising in peak temperatures on hot days.

1 SUNDAY

WHY I SUPPORT BREAST CANCER TRIALS

My first thought was of my children – they need me and I have to get through this for them. Clinical trials are a beacon of hope. Every breakthrough exists because someone before us was willing to participate in research, and by supporting clinical trials, we are paying that gift forward.

Julie Simms, diagnosed age 43

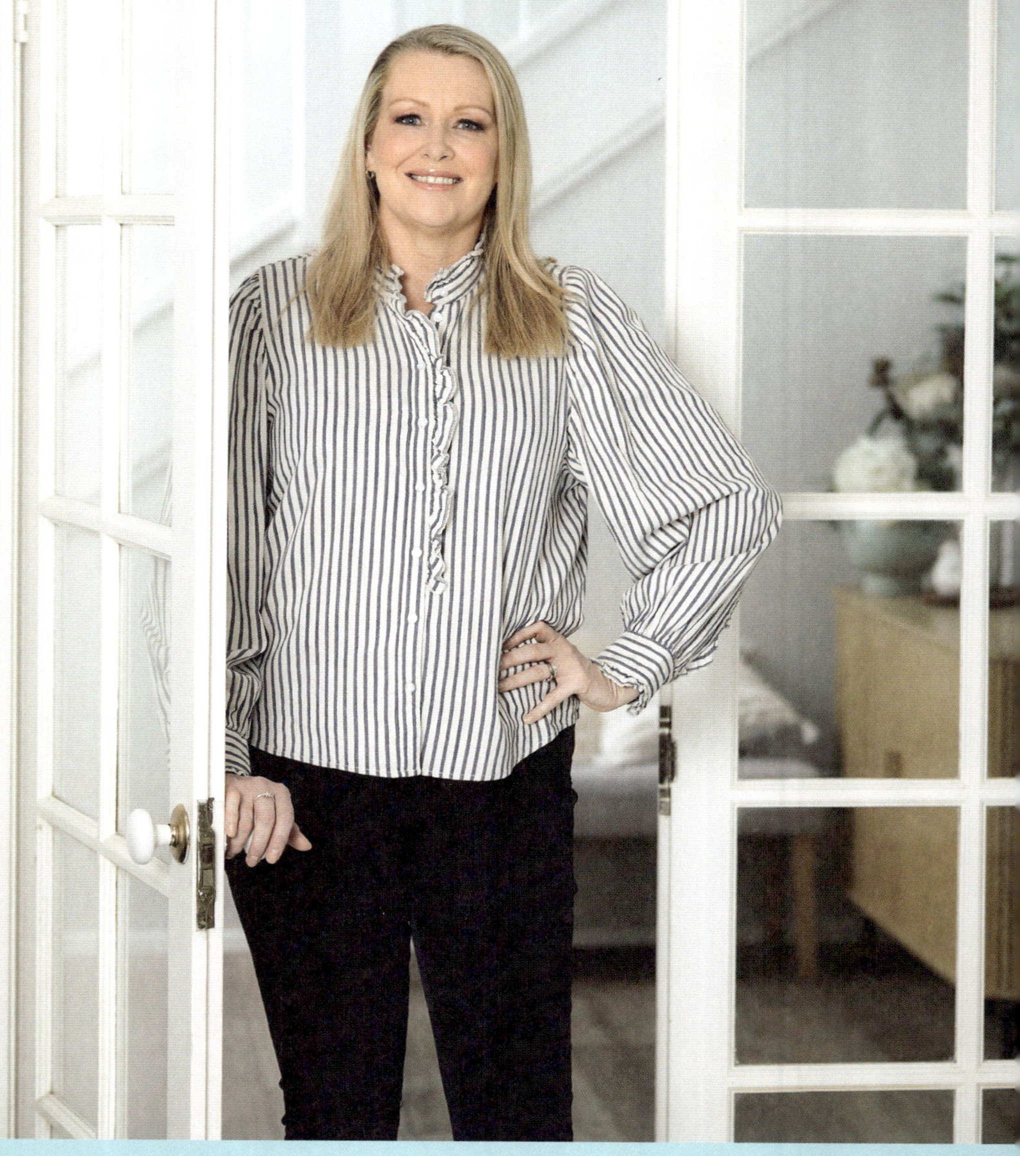

let's talk about NUTRITION

Following a healthy, balanced diet is the key to good nutrition. With tips from this chapter, you can fuel your body, protect yourself from illness and disease and find new ways to enjoy your daily meals.

Do you find yourself reaching for the chocolate when you need a pick-me-up, skipping lunch when you're busy or snacking on chips before bedtime? Over time, these habits can lead to weight loss or gain, tooth decay, low mood, fatigue and an increased risk of heart disease and diabetes. In good news, small changes over time can help create new habits to replace the unhelpful ones. Here's how.

HABIT #1 Skipping meals
Busyness, forgetfulness or poor time management might mean you're not eating for long periods of time, which can impair concentration, disrupt blood glucose levels, slow the metabolism and lead to increased anxiety or disordered eating.
Try this: Block out time to eat at regular intervals, and keep quick and easy options on hand if motivation is stopping you. If you don't have the appetite for large meals, enjoy smaller meals or snacks every few hours.

HABIT #2 Emotional eating
Fifty-five per cent of Australians admit they turn to food when they feel depressed or stressed, with chocolate, chips and biscuits popular choices. While this habit isn't inherently harmful, it could lead to weight gain, binge eating or feelings of guilt or shame.

Try this: Identify your stress triggers and look for non-food-related ways to combat them – for example, taking a walk, calling a friend or having a hot shower. Be kind to yourself and remember, tomorrow is a new day.

HABIT #3 Snacking before bedtime
You're a regular late-night fridge-raider, snacking on less-than-ideal options like chips, chocolate or ice cream before bed.
Try this: New research shows having a light snack before bedtime can be beneficial for sleep and helps stabilise blood glucose levels for those with diabetes. The trick is to choose healthy options like a piece of fruit, a handful of nuts, a cup of herbal tea or a glass of milk.

HABIT #4 Convenience over nutrition
Our increasingly busy lives see us resorting to takeaway and processed foods more and more. Unfortunately, these options are sometimes high in salt and saturated fats, which can contribute to weight gain, heart disease, bowel irregularities and diabetes.
Try this: Plan out your meals for the week and do some preparation ahead of time, so you have healthy options on hand for those days when you don't have the time or energy to cook. Give yourself a night off by utilising meal delivery services with a health focus, such as Lite n' Easy or HelloFresh.

For more information, visit Nutrition Australia; nutritionaustralia.org

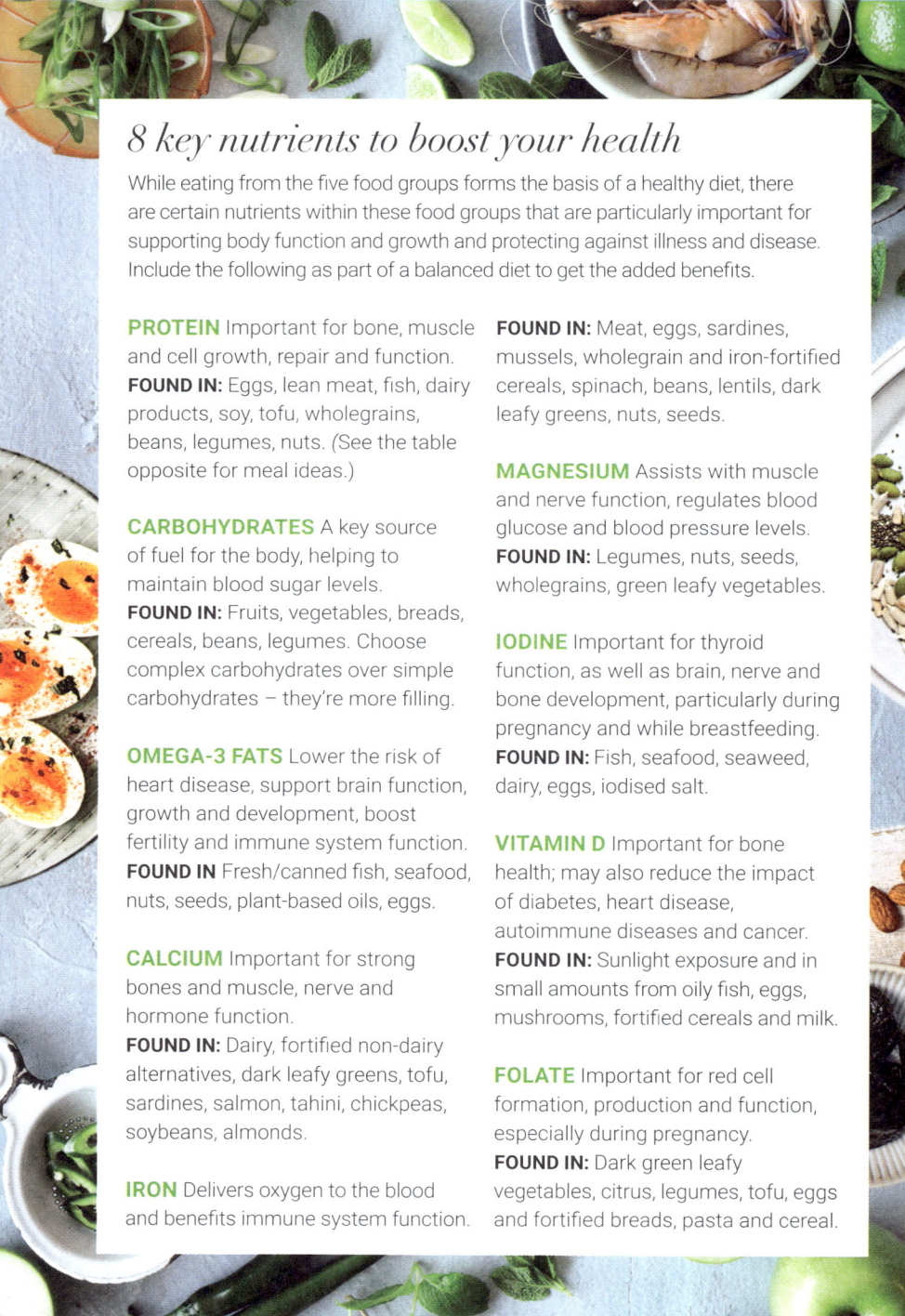

8 key nutrients to boost your health

While eating from the five food groups forms the basis of a healthy diet, there are certain nutrients within these food groups that are particularly important for supporting body function and growth and protecting against illness and disease. Include the following as part of a balanced diet to get the added benefits.

PROTEIN Important for bone, muscle and cell growth, repair and function.
FOUND IN: Eggs, lean meat, fish, dairy products, soy, tofu, wholegrains, beans, legumes, nuts. (See the table opposite for meal ideas.)

CARBOHYDRATES A key source of fuel for the body, helping to maintain blood sugar levels.
FOUND IN: Fruits, vegetables, breads, cereals, beans, legumes. Choose complex carbohydrates over simple carbohydrates – they're more filling.

OMEGA-3 FATS Lower the risk of heart disease, support brain function, growth and development, boost fertility and immune system function.
FOUND IN Fresh/canned fish, seafood, nuts, seeds, plant-based oils, eggs.

CALCIUM Important for strong bones and muscle, nerve and hormone function.
FOUND IN: Dairy, fortified non-dairy alternatives, dark leafy greens, tofu, sardines, salmon, tahini, chickpeas, soybeans, almonds.

IRON Delivers oxygen to the blood and benefits immune system function.
FOUND IN: Meat, eggs, sardines, mussels, wholegrain and iron-fortified cereals, spinach, beans, lentils, dark leafy greens, nuts, seeds.

MAGNESIUM Assists with muscle and nerve function, regulates blood glucose and blood pressure levels.
FOUND IN: Legumes, nuts, seeds, wholegrains, green leafy vegetables.

IODINE Important for thyroid function, as well as brain, nerve and bone development, particularly during pregnancy and while breastfeeding.
FOUND IN: Fish, seafood, seaweed, dairy, eggs, iodised salt.

VITAMIN D Important for bone health; may also reduce the impact of diabetes, heart disease, autoimmune diseases and cancer.
FOUND IN: Sunlight exposure and in small amounts from oily fish, eggs, mushrooms, fortified cereals and milk.

FOLATE Important for red cell formation, production and function, especially during pregnancy.
FOUND IN: Dark green leafy vegetables, citrus, legumes, tofu, eggs and fortified breads, pasta and cereal.

Protein-rich meal ideas

Adding protein to your diet can have a host of benefits, including building muscle, increasing energy levels and assisting with weight loss. Australian women should consume at least 0.8-1 gram of protein per kilogram of body weight each day (for example, a 60 kilogram woman needs 50-60 grams). Meet your requirements with these protein-packed meal ideas.

BREAKFAST

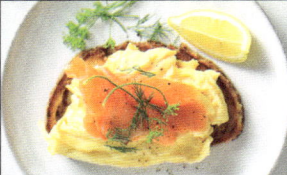 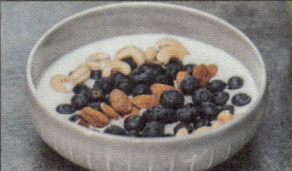 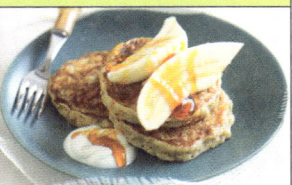

SCRAMBLED EGGS Whisk eggs with cheese and cook until just set. Serve on wholegrain toast with smoked salmon or spinach.

GREEK YOGHURT Quick and simple, serve a bowl of Greek yoghurt topped with berries, nuts and seeds (try cashews, almonds or chia seeds).

PROTEIN PANCAKES Make a batch of pancakes using eggs, oat or wholemeal flour and milk. Top with banana, peanut butter and yoghurt.

LUNCH

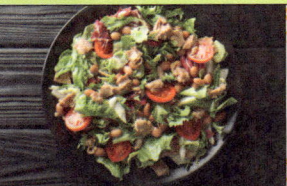 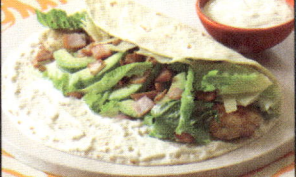 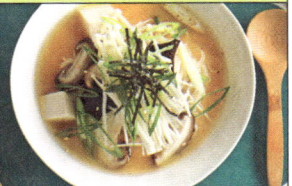

TUNA SALAD Fill your plate with leafy greens then top with a can of tuna or a boiled egg, canned beans, tomatoes and a drizzle of olive oil.

CHICKEN WRAP Make a portable lunch by filling a wholemeal wrap with cooked chicken, avocado, salad and hummus or cottage cheese.

MISO SOUP Prepare a broth from miso paste and water and add extra protein with tofu, mushrooms, soba noodles or edamame.

DINNER

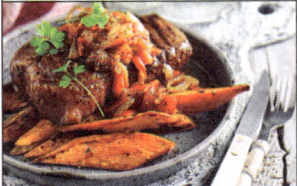 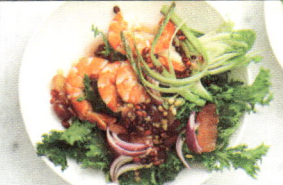 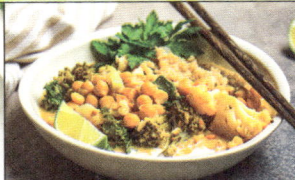

STEAK AND CHIPS Cook a piece of lean beef or pork on the barbecue and serve with a side of oven-baked sweet potato chips or asparagus.

PRAWN SALAD For summer nights, make a salad of green leafy vegetables, cooked prawns, avocado and a zesty lime olive oil dressing.

CHICKPEA CURRY Make a curry with chickpeas, coconut milk, cauliflower and spinach; lentils work well, too. Serve with brown rice.

Navigating dietary requirements

People can have a restricted diet for medical, health, cultural or personal reasons. Familiarise yourself with their needs and follow this guide when preparing food for them.

1. **Ask lots of questions** Plan ahead and ask guests or family members if they have any dietary needs, allergies or personal preferences. If you're a guest at someone's home, mention your needs (or your child's) to your host and offer to bring some suitable foods.

2. **Be inclusive** Rather than making one separate meal for the person with dietary needs, plan a menu of dishes that everyone will enjoy. Proteins and sides can be cooked separately, with sauces or dressings served on the side.

3. **Minimise cross contamination** Before you start cooking, thoroughly clean all food preparation areas, chopping boards, knives and spoons, and allocate separate utensils for any allergenic foods. Cook and store foods separately so there's no risk of an allergen making its way into the wrong dish.

4. **Keep it stress-free** If in doubt, utilise ready-made supermarket products tailored to dietary requirements. They are produced in commercial kitchens to strict conditions. Read labels carefully and choose options without too many additives or artificial ingredients.

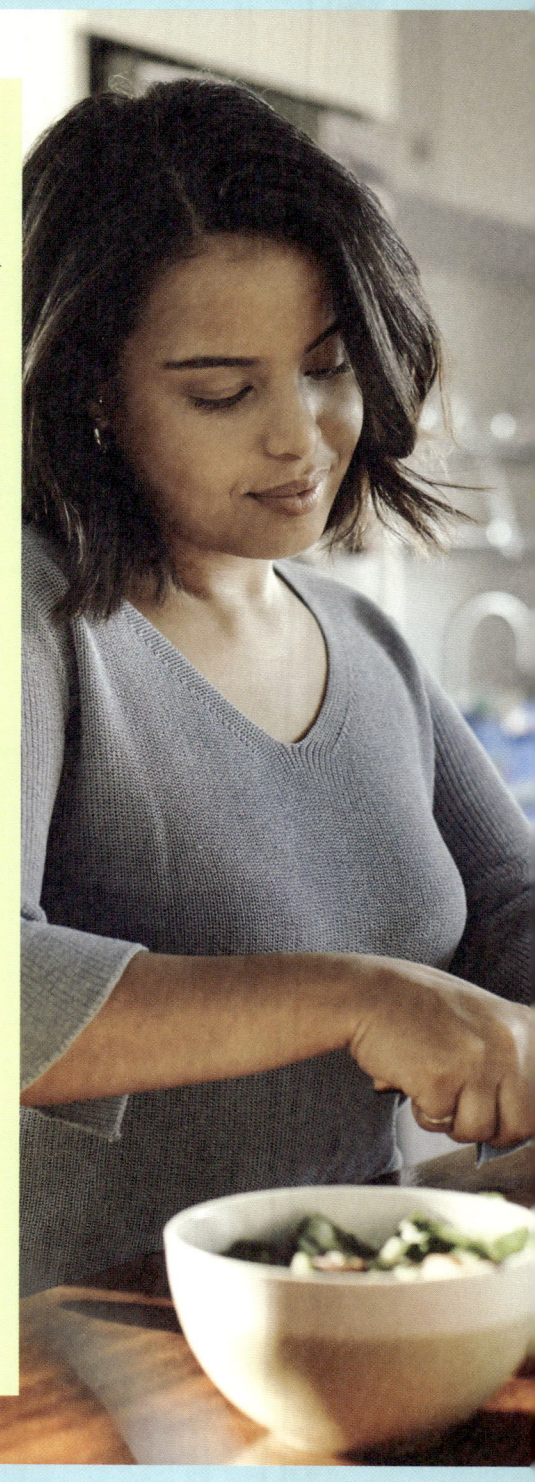

COMMON DIETARY REQUIREMENTS EXPLAINED
Understand family and friends' needs and swap out ingredients with this guide.

LACTOSE INTOLERANCE
Avoid Milk, cheese, butter, cream, ice cream, prepared cake mixes and baked goods, cream-based sauces, processed meats, some confectionery.
Substitute Lactose-free, rice, oat, almond, coconut or soy milks and products.

COELIAC DISEASE (gluten intolerance)
Avoid Foods containing gluten and made from wheat, barley, oats or rye, including bread, pasta, cereals, crackers, baked goods, beer and many processed foods.
Substitute Gluten-free grains and flours, rice, quinoa, corn, tapioca, buckwheat, lentils and chickpeas (check product labels).

DIABETES
Avoid Foods high in added sugar, sodium or trans fats, refined carbohydrates.
Substitute Low-glycaemic index foods, like wholegrains, legumes, fruit, vegetables, lean protein and low-fat dairy.

VEGETARIANISM
Avoid Meat, poultry, fish and seafood, and in some cases, eggs and dairy.
Substitute Plant-based proteins, such as pulses, legumes and soy-derived products, such as tofu or tempeh.

VEGANISM
Avoid All animal-derived foods, including meat, seafood, milk products, fish-derived sauces, honey, eggs, gelatin and whey.
Substitute Wholegrains, fruits, vegetables, legumes, seeds, rice malt or maple syrup.

HALAL
Avoid Pork and pork products, meat from animals not slaughtered according to Islamic law and any food product prepared using alcohol, animal shortening, lard, gelatin or vanilla extract (pure or artificial).
Substitute A vegetarian alternative or foods that are certified Halal.

KOSHER
Avoid Meat products from non-Kosher animals, including pork, rabbit, camel, kangaroo, cuts of beef from the hindquarters and shellfish. Meat and dairy should not be served at the same time and there are additional restrictions during Passover.
Substitute Kosher-certified protein, as well as fish, eggs, fruit, vegetables and grains.

FOOD ALLERGIES
Avoid All traces of the allergy-causing ingredient, such as wheat, nuts, cow's milk, egg, fish, shellfish and soy.

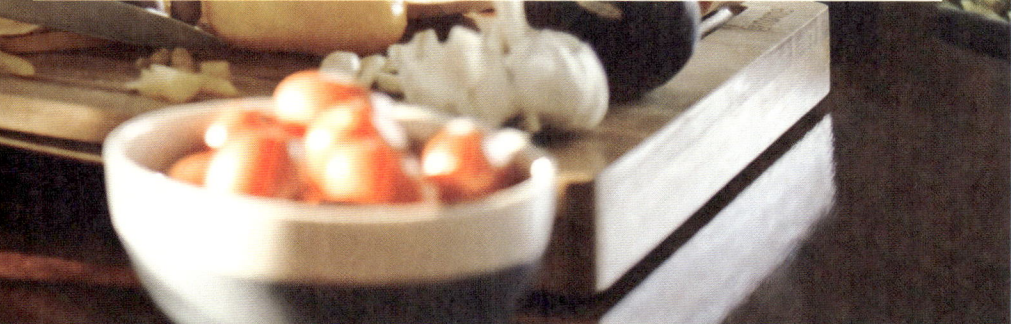

	FEBRUARY					
S	M	T	W	T	F	S
	1	2	3	4	5	6	7
8	9	10	11	12	13	14
15	16	17	18	19	20	21
22	23	24	25	26	27	28

	MARCH					
S	M	T	W	T	F	S
1	2	3	4	5	6	7
8	9	10	11	12	13	14
15	16	17	18	19	20	21
22	23	24	25	26	27	28
29	30	31				

	APRIL					
S	M	T	W	T	F	S
			1	2	3	4
5	6	7	8	9	10	11
12	13	14	15	16	17	18
19	20	21	22	23	24	25
26	27	28	29	30		

2 MONDAY LABOUR DAY (WA)

3 TUESDAY

4 WEDNESDAY HOLI (HINDU FESTIVAL)

5 THURSDAY

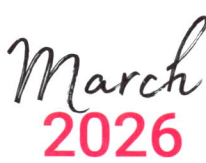
March 2026

6 FRIDAY

7 SATURDAY

REDUCE YOUR SALT INTAKE by opting for low-sodium versions of canned goods, sauces and processed foods, and flavouring meals with herbs and spices.

8 SUNDAY INTERNATIONAL WOMEN'S DAY

	FEBRUARY					
S	M	T	W	T	F	S
1	2	3	4	5	6	7
8	9	10	11	12	13	14
15	16	17	18	19	20	21
22	23	24	25	26	27	28

	MARCH					
S	M	T	W	T	F	S
1	2	3	4	5	6	7
8	9	10	11	12	13	14
15	16	17	18	19	20	21
22	23	24	25	26	27	28
29	30	31				

	APRIL					
S	M	T	W	T	F	S
			1	2	3	4
5	6	7	8	9	10	11
12	13	14	15	16	17	18
19	20	21	22	23	24	25
26	27	28	29	30		

9 MONDAY LABOUR DAY (VIC), EIGHT HOURS DAY (TAS), ADELAIDE CUP (SA), CANBERRA DAY (ACT)

10 TUESDAY

11 WEDNESDAY

12 THURSDAY

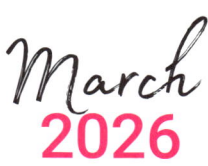

March 2026

13 FRIDAY

14 SATURDAY

HELP ENSURE THIS DIARY IS RELEVANT to you by taking our survey at breastcancertrials.org.au/VIPDiaryOffer. You'll unlock a special offer as our thanks.

15 SUNDAY

	FEBRUARY					
S	M	T	W	T	F	S
	1	2	3	4	5	6	7
8	9	10	11	12	13	14
15	16	17	18	19	20	21
22	23	24	25	26	27	28

	MARCH					
S	M	T	W	T	F	S
1	2	3	4	5	6	7
8	9	10	11	12	13	14
15	16	17	18	19	20	21
22	23	24	25	26	27	28
29	30	31				

	APRIL					
S	M	T	W	T	F	S
			1	2	3	4
5	6	7	8	9	10	11
12	13	14	15	16	17	18
19	20	21	22	23	24	25
26	27	28	29	30		

16 MONDAY

17 TUESDAY ST PATRICK'S DAY

18 WEDNESDAY

19 THURSDAY NATIONAL CLOSE THE GAP DAY

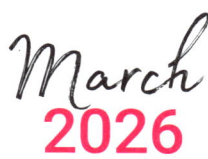
March
2026

20 FRIDAY EID AL-FITR (ISLAMIC HOLIDAY)

21 SATURDAY HARMONY DAY, NOWRUZ (PERSIAN NEW YEAR)

> **ADD SOME PLANT-BASED MEALS** to your repertoire as a nutritious and inexpensive option. Think vegetable soups, curries, pizzas, salads and bean burgers.

22 SUNDAY

		FEB	RUA	RY		
S	M	T	W	T	F	S
1	2	3	4	5	6	7
8	9	10	11	12	13	14
15	16	17	18	19	20	21
22	23	24	25	26	27	28

		MA	RC	H		
S	M	T	W	T	F	S
1	2	3	4	5	6	7
8	9	10	11	12	13	14
15	16	17	18	19	20	21
22	23	24	25	26	27	28
29	30	31				

		AP	RI	L		
S	M	T	W	T	F	S
			1	2	3	4
5	6	7	8	9	10	11
12	13	14	15	16	17	18
19	20	21	22	23	24	25
26	27	28	29	30		

23 MONDAY

24 TUESDAY

25 WEDNESDAY

26 THURSDAY

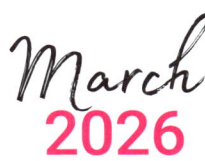
March 2026

27 FRIDAY

28 SATURDAY

> **BE A SAVVY SHOPPER** by reading nutrition panels and ingredients lists on products. Avoid items that are high in sugar, salt or unhealthy fats, and check for allergen statements.

29 SUNDAY PALM SUNDAY

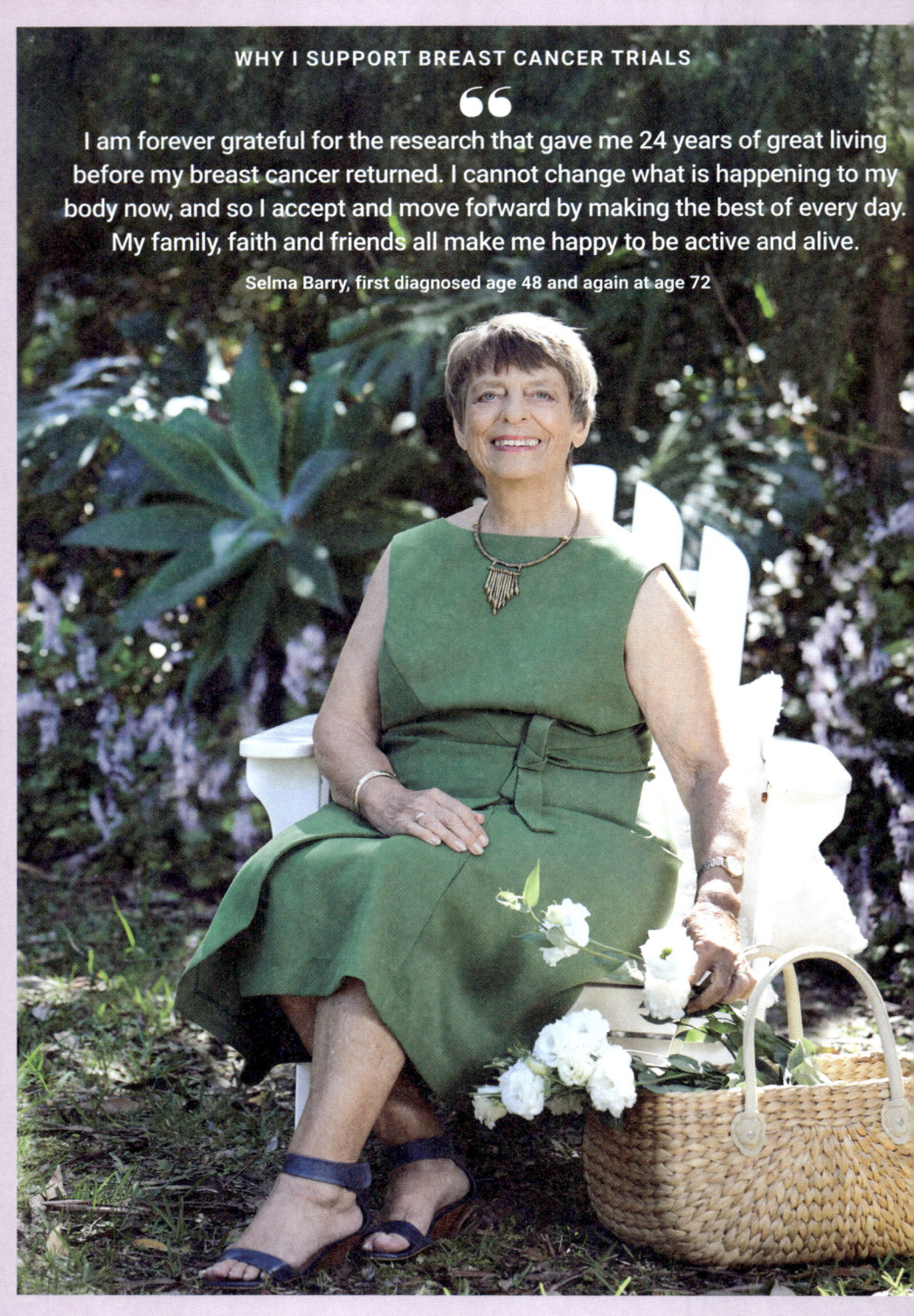

WHY I SUPPORT BREAST CANCER TRIALS

> I am forever grateful for the research that gave me 24 years of great living before my breast cancer returned. I cannot change what is happening to my body now, and so I accept and move forward by making the best of every day. My family, faith and friends all make me happy to be active and alive.

Selma Barry, first diagnosed age 48 and again at age 72

let's talk about
WOMEN'S HEALTH

The demands of being a mother, daughter, partner and employee often see women neglecting their own health. Take back control by reading up on the conditions and issues that affect you.

Currently, one in three Australians hold a negative bias based on gender. Nearly half of the world's population think that men make better political leaders than women while gender non-binary people are more likely to experience prejudice than men and women. These outdated views of a person's capabilities and social rights based on their gender can limit opportunities and have far-reaching effects on a person's safety, mental wellbeing and financial capabilities.

WHAT IS GENDER BIAS?
Gender bias is the act of giving preferential treatment to one gender over another. This bias and inequality is prevalent in every aspect of our lives. At school, children might be steered towards certain subjects or activities or feel pressure to conform to gender stereotypes. In the workplace, women are often paid less than their male counterparts and may not have access to the same training or career progression. At home, gender bias can be subtle, such as household jobs being divvied up based on gender or women taking on the unpaid care of children. In some cases, these biases may contribute to domestic violence, sexual assault or financial abuse.

TACKLING GENDER BIAS AT HOME
- Check the distribution of domestic duties in your household – are roles like cooking or mowing the lawn evenly split across genders?
- Share parenting responsibilities, including drop-offs, homework, laundry, meal preparation and school events.
- Encourage emotional expression and physical affection in children of all genders, teaching empathy and kindness to others.
- Give children opportunities based on their interests – sport, music, coding and dance are not gender exclusive. Similarly, as an adult, don't be afraid to choose hobbies that have been traditionally geared towards the opposite gender.
- Seek out mixed-gender social groups, sporting teams or activities and enjoy friendships with all gender identities. Share your views and challenge ideas that may be harmful or belittling to others.
- Be conscious of your language. Avoid praising people on their physical appearance or attributes and try to use gender-neutral terms for professions, such as firefighter instead of fireman or flight attendant rather than stewardess.
- Have open discussions with your family around gendered marketing or outdated gender stereotypes in TV shows and movies, and why they're not OK.

For more information, visit Working for Women; genderequality.gov.au

5 ways to take care of your gut

Did you know there are trillions of bacteria, fungi, viruses and parasites living in your gastrointestinal system, which includes the stomach, intestines and colon – aka your gut? The gut microbiome plays an important role in your digestive health and other areas like the immune system. When it's out of balance, you may experience gut-related issues, such as irritable bowel syndrome, bloating, cramping, constipation or diarrhoea. Women are particularly susceptible during menstruation, pregnancy and menopause, when our hormones fluctuate; anxiety and stress can also exacerbate gut problems. Take special care of your gut health with these steps.

1 Go for a walk
Exercise enhances the number and variety of beneficial microbiome in our bodies, and walking is particularly beneficial. A short stroll after meals can help with the digestive process as well as blood-sugar management.

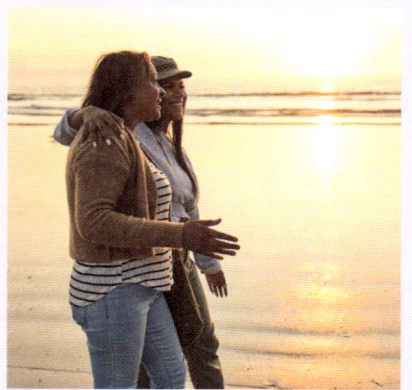

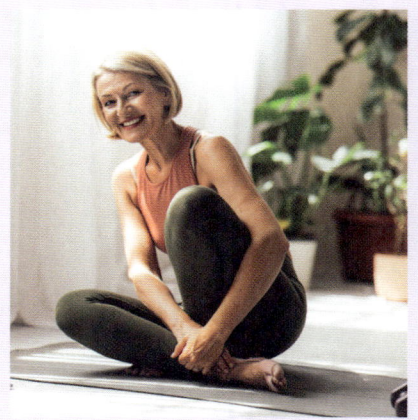

2 Manage anxiety
People with irritable bowel syndrome have a higher risk of depression and anxiety than those without. Consider yoga, meditation, breathing exercises or mind-body therapies like cognitive behavioural therapy to calm the mind and manage anxious thoughts.

3 Keep a gut diary
If you often suffer from gut-related issues, it's a good idea to keep track of the events surrounding their occurrence. Write down what you eat and drink, how much sleep you're getting, your exercise habits and any triggers that may affect your mood to give your GP some insight into what could be causing your gut issues.

4 Prioritise sleep
Sleep plays an important role in immune function, weight and overall health, so aim for seven to nine hours each night. To aid in this, create a wind-down routine without screens and keep your bedroom dark and cool.

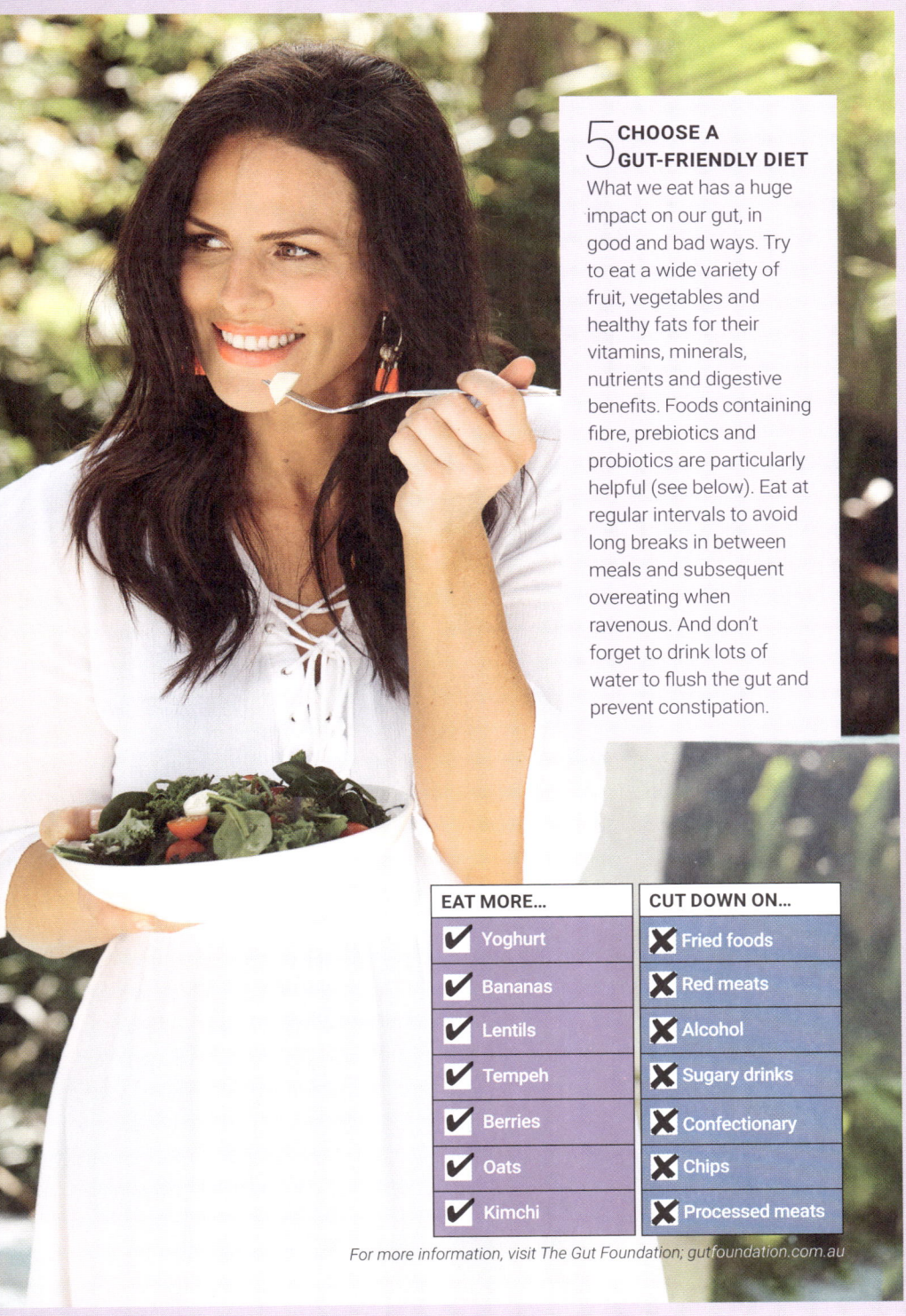

5 CHOOSE A GUT-FRIENDLY DIET

What we eat has a huge impact on our gut, in good and bad ways. Try to eat a wide variety of fruit, vegetables and healthy fats for their vitamins, minerals, nutrients and digestive benefits. Foods containing fibre, prebiotics and probiotics are particularly helpful (see below). Eat at regular intervals to avoid long breaks in between meals and subsequent overeating when ravenous. And don't forget to drink lots of water to flush the gut and prevent constipation.

EAT MORE...	CUT DOWN ON...
✔ Yoghurt	✘ Fried foods
✔ Bananas	✘ Red meats
✔ Lentils	✘ Alcohol
✔ Tempeh	✘ Sugary drinks
✔ Berries	✘ Confectionary
✔ Oats	✘ Chips
✔ Kimchi	✘ Processed meats

For more information, visit The Gut Foundation; gutfoundation.com.au

Navigating perimenopause

THE FACTS
When you reach your 40s, you'll likely enter a new stage of life called perimenopause. Lasting anywhere from one to 10 years, this is when your body transitions to the end of its reproductive phase. Irregular periods are a common sign of perimenopause, and you may also experience other physical, emotional and mental symptoms. Perimenopause ends 12 months after the date of your last period, at which point you enter menopause. Follow these steps to navigate this necessary time of change.

MANAGE SYMPTOMS
The hormonal fluctuations of perimenopause can cause hot flushes and night sweats, disturbed sleep, muscle and joint soreness, vaginal dryness, sore breasts, mood swings, brain fog, anxiety, depression and weight gain. For some women, these are mild, but for others they can be severe. Seek treatment if symptoms are bothering you or impacting your life. Your doctor may recommend menopausal hormone therapy (MHT), non-hormonal medicines, cognitive behavioural therapy or practical measures, such as wearing layers and natural fibres.

TWEAK YOUR LIFESTYLE
Giving up smoking comes with a long list of health benefits and can lessen the effects of hot flushes, eating a healthy diet can help with weight gain and regular exercise is hugely beneficial for boosting mood. Mindfulness, meditation, massage and sleep are all wonderful for relieving stress.

CONTINUE WITH CONTRACEPTION
You can still fall pregnant while going through perimenopause, so keep up with your chosen form of contraception for at least one year after your last menstrual period if you don't plan on having children.

SEEK SUPPORT
Every woman's menopausal experience will be different, so you need a treatment plan tailored to your individual symptoms and circumstances. Along with your GP, consider seeing a counsellor or psychologist for emotional support, as well as confiding in your partner and close friends.

EMBRACE THE CHANGE
Perimenopause usually coincides with mid-life. See this as an opportunity to invest in you. Buy yourself a new wardrobe (you'll want light layers and natural fibres), plan a trip to a bucket-list destination or take up a new hobby.

For more information, visit the Australasian Menopause Society; menopause.org.au

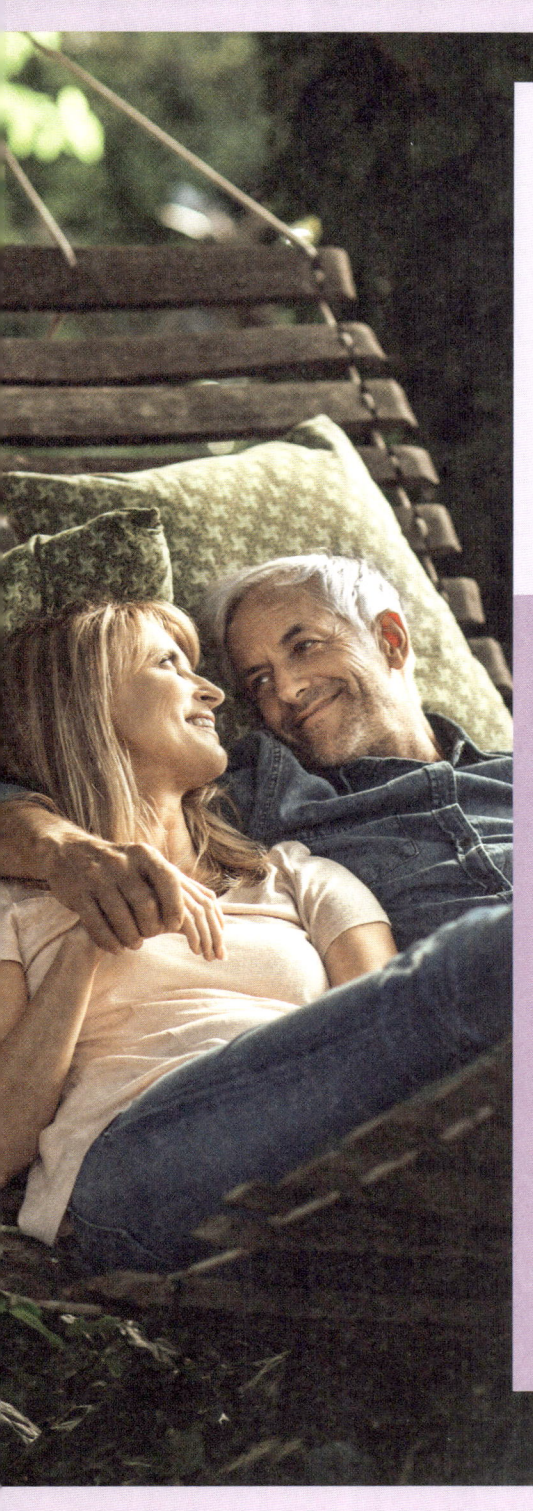

Simple tricks to boost your sex drive

A woman's libido – that is her desire to engage in sexual activity – can vary greatly through life. There is no 'normal' level – some people feel like having sex every day while others rarely have the desire. A drop in libido can be due to shifting hormone levels, physical changes, body image, lack of intimacy or stress. There is no need to worry unless your sex drive bothers you or causes problems in your relationship. If so, try the following.

TRY THESE TIPS TO GIVE YOUR LIBIDO A BOOST

Seek counselling or advice from a GP, psychologist or hormone specialist to address any physical or relationship issues.

Enjoy regular exercise to increase stamina, improve body image and lift your mood.

Reduce habits that can dampen sexual desire, such as smoking, drinking alcohol or taking drugs.

Manage stress associated with work, finances or children, which may be impacting your sex drive. Try journalling, meditation or make time for self-care.

Schedule intimacy into your calendar. It may not seem very romantic, but planning regular one-on-one time can help shift your libido in the right direction.

Talk with your partner to build a stronger emotional connection. Speak openly about your likes and dislikes in the bedroom.

		MARCH				
S	M	T	W	T	F	S
1	2	3	4	5	6	7
8	9	10	11	12	13	14
15	16	17	18	19	20	21
22	23	24	25	26	27	28
29	30	31				

		APRIL				
S	M	T	W	T	F	S
			1	2	3	4
5	6	7	8	9	10	11
12	13	14	15	16	17	18
19	20	21	22	23	24	25
26	27	28	29	30		

		MAY				
S	M	T	W	T	F	S
31					1	2
3	4	5	6	7	8	9
10	11	12	13	14	15	16
17	18	19	20	21	22	23
24	25	26	27	28	29	30

30 MONDAY

31 TUESDAY

1 WEDNESDAY

2 THURSDAY PASSOVER BEGINS

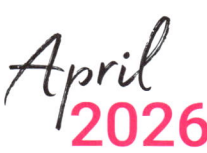
April 2026

3 FRIDAY GOOD FRIDAY

4 SATURDAY

> **AIM TO EAT AT THE SAME TIMES EACH DAY** to help promote optimal digestion, regulate hunger hormones and avoid bloating and discomfort.

5 SUNDAY EASTER SUNDAY, DAYLIGHT SAVING TIME ENDS (ACT, NSW, SA, TAS, VIC)

		MARCH				
S	M	T	W	T	F	S
	2	3	4	5	6	7
8	9	10	11	12	13	14
15	16	17	18	19	20	21
22	23	24	25	26	27	28
29	30	31				

		APRIL				
S	M	T	W	T	F	S
			1	2	3	4
5	6	7	8	9	10	11
12	13	14	15	16	17	18
19	20	21	22	23	24	25
26	27	28	29	30		

		MAY				
S	M	T	W	T	F	S
31					1	2
3	4	5	6	7	8	9
10	11	12	13	14	15	16
17	18	19	20	21	22	23
24	25	26	27	28	29	30

6 MONDAY   EASTER MONDAY

7 TUESDAY   EASTER TUESDAY (TAS)

8 WEDNESDAY

9 THURSDAY

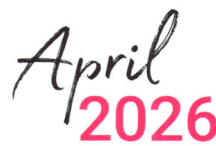

April 2026

10 FRIDAY

11 SATURDAY

> **PERIOD PAIN IS NORMAL TO A POINT,** but see your doctor if menstrual symptoms are causing you to miss school, work or social events.

12 SUNDAY ORTHODOX EASTER

	MARCH					
S	M	T	W	T	F	S
1	2	3	4	5	6	7
8	9	10	11	12	13	14
15	16	17	18	19	20	21
22	23	24	25	26	27	28
29	30	31				

	APRIL					
S	M	T	W	T	F	S
			1	2	3	4
5	6	7	8	9	10	11
12	13	14	15	16	17	18
19	20	21	22	23	24	25
26	27	28	29	30		

	MAY					
S	M	T	W	T	F	S
31					1	2
3	4	5	6	7	8	9
10	11	12	13	14	15	16
17	18	19	20	21	22	23
24	25	26	27	28	29	30

13 MONDAY

14 TUESDAY

15 WEDNESDAY

16 THURSDAY

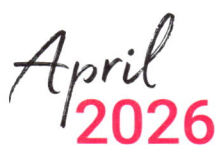
April 2026

17 FRIDAY

18 SATURDAY

STAY INFORMED of the latest breast cancer research by signing up to the Breast Cancer Trials e-newsletter. Visit breastcancertrials.org.au/e-news-signup.

19 SUNDAY

		MARCH				
S	M	T	W	T	F	S
1	2	3	4	5	6	7
8	9	10	11	12	13	14
15	16	17	18	19	20	21
22	23	24	25	26	27	28
29	30	31				

		APRIL				
S	M	T	W	T	F	S
			1	2	3	4
5	6	7	8	9	10	11
12	13	14	15	16	17	18
19	20	21	22	23	24	25
26	27	28	29	30		

		MAY				
S	M	T	W	T	F	S
31					1	2
3	4	5	6	7	8	9
10	11	12	13	14	15	16
17	18	19	20	21	22	23
24	25	26	27	28	29	30

20 MONDAY

21 TUESDAY

22 WEDNESDAY

23 THURSDAY

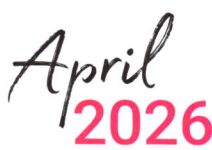

April 2026

24 FRIDAY

25 SATURDAY <small>ANZAC DAY</small>

> **REDUCE THE STIGMA AROUND GUT HEALTH** by having open and honest conversations with your friends, family and most importantly, your GP.

26 SUNDAY

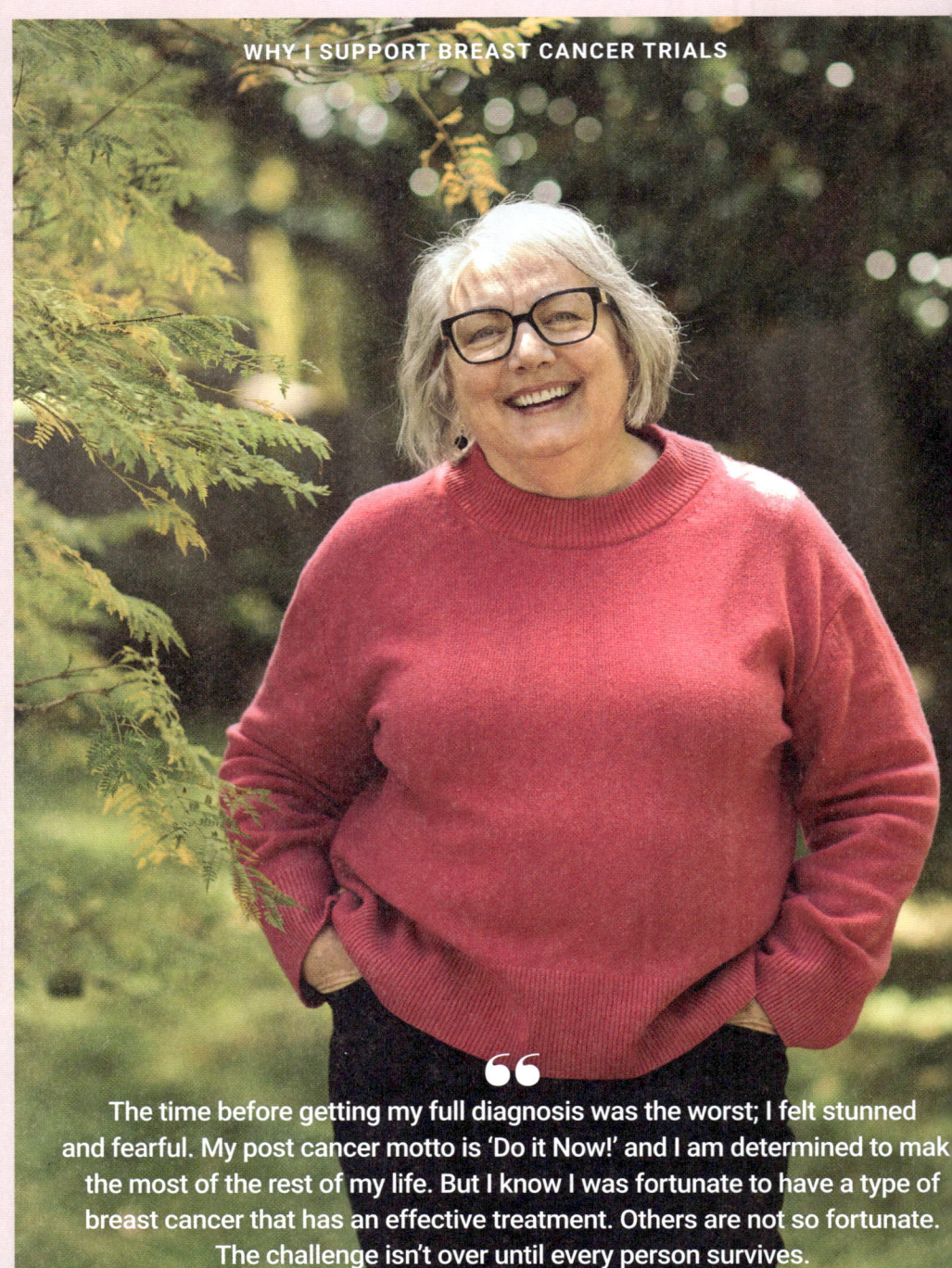

WHY I SUPPORT BREAST CANCER TRIALS

> The time before getting my full diagnosis was the worst; I felt stunned and fearful. My post cancer motto is 'Do it Now!' and I am determined to make the most of the rest of my life. But I know I was fortunate to have a type of breast cancer that has an effective treatment. Others are not so fortunate. The challenge isn't over until every person survives.

Merryn Carter, diagnosed age 52

let's talk about HEART HEALTH

Cardiovascular disease kills one woman almost every hour of every day in Australia. Our risk changes with age, so it's important to be aware of the symptoms and lifestyle changes that could save your life.

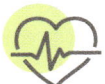

Heart disease and breast cancer are among the top five causes of death for Australian women, and they also share another link. While breast cancer survival rates have improved significantly over the last 30 years, those same survivors are at an increased risk of cardiovascular complications, including heart failure, heart attack and high blood pressure.

HOW CAN BREAST CANCER AFFECT YOUR HEART?

Several factors can increase a breast cancer survivor's risk of cardiovascular disease.

Treatments – Some breast cancer treatments, such as radiation therapy and some chemotherapy drugs, can cause cardiotoxicity – damage or dysfunction of the heart muscle related to cancer treatment. While rare, cancer treatment can sometimes cause heart failure.

Common risk factors – Heart disease and breast cancer share some risk factors, such as obesity, physical inactivity, poor diet and smoking. Having one or more risk factors may increase your risk for both conditions.

Hormonal factors – Oestrogen has the potential to affect the cardiovascular system as well as act to stimulate breast cancer growth. When women undergo hormonal therapy for breast cancer, it can also increase their cholesterol levels and blood pressure, contributing to cardiovascular complications.

MANAGEMENT AND PREVENTION STRATEGIES

- Recognise the signs of cardiotoxicity for early intervention. Seek medical advice for shortness of breath, chest pain or discomfort, fatigue, swelling and irregular heartbeat. Most side effects show up in the first 12 months after treatment, although some may occur later in life.
- Make lifestyle changes to reduce your risk of both diseases. Quit smoking, follow a heart-healthy diet, enjoy regular moderate exercise and take steps to reduce stress.
- Stay on top of heart checks to monitor and manage your blood pressure, cholesterol levels and blood glucose levels.
- Keep in regular contact with your healthcare team, and join breast cancer support groups or survivorship programs to access valuable resources and emotional support.

> *Cancer survivors are up to eight times more likely to develop cardiovascular disease as a result of their treatment.*

For more information, visit Breast Cancer Trials; breastcancertrials.org.au

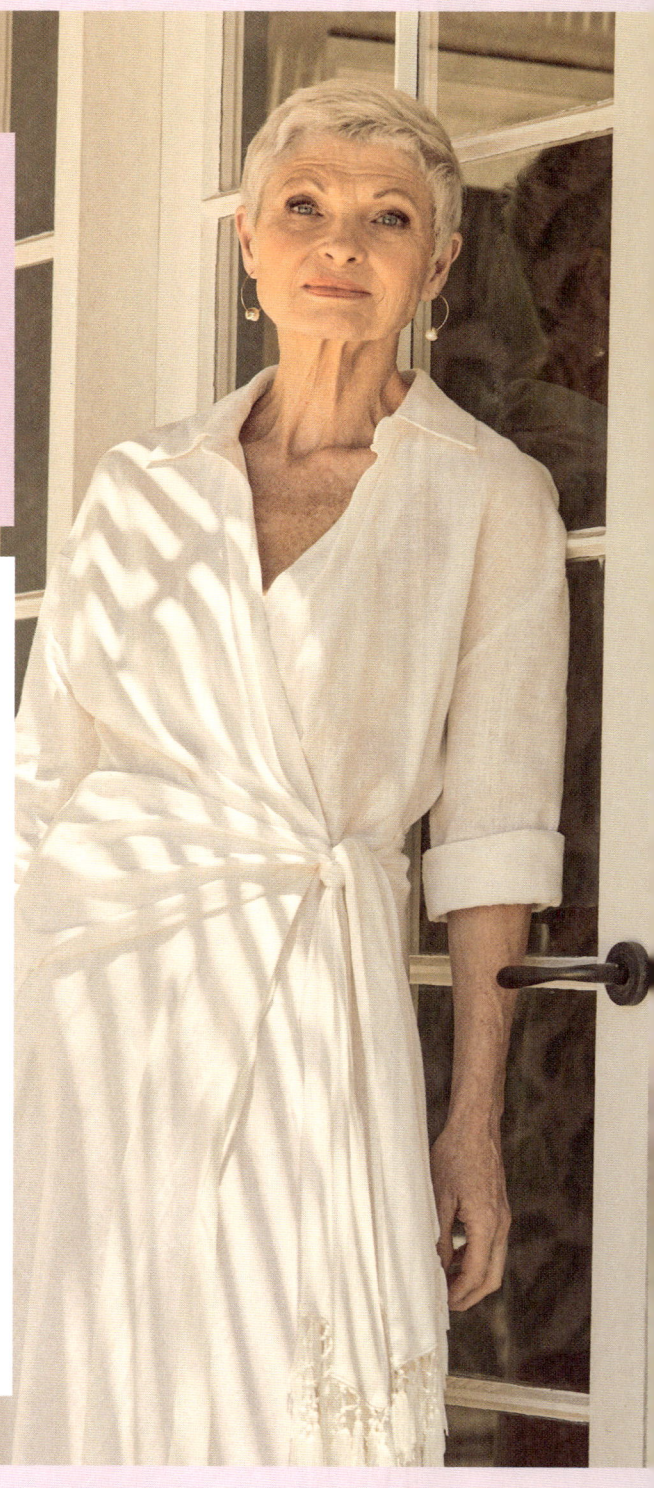

KNOW YOUR HEART DISEASE RISK

Along with the traditional heart disease risk factors, women have their own set of additional risk factors. Some we can change, others we can't. Get to know the risks below, then see the opposite page for ways to manage them.

RISK FACTORS YOU CAN MODIFY

High cholesterol

High blood pressure

Obesity

Diabetes

Stress and depression

Smoking

Inactivity

Poor diet

UNMODIFIABLE RISK FACTORS

Age

Menopause

Pregnancy complications (preeclampsia, gestational diabetes)

Family history

8 essentials for heart health

1 Healthy diet
Eat plenty of fruit, vegetables, wholegrains and healthy protein-rich foods (such as fish, eggs, lean poultry or plant-based options like legumes, nuts and seeds), limiting red meat to one to three times a week. Also include milk, yoghurt or cheese and healthy fats like avocado, olive oil, nuts and seeds. Use herbs and spices in place of salt to flavour food.

2 Exercise
Aim to enjoy at least 30 minutes of vigorous activity each day. This can be split across the day and includes intermittent activity like playing with pets, carrying shopping bags, climbing stairs or walking to the bus stop.

3 Quit smoking
Make a quit plan and discuss strategies with your GP, contact Quitline on 13 QUIT (137 848) or via quit.org.au and seek support from friends and loved ones.

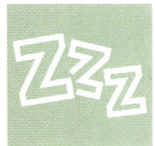

4 Sleep
Adults should aim to get seven to nine hours of sleep each night to protect your heart. Maintaining regular sleep and wake times, avoiding caffeine or alcohol in the hours before bed and introducing wind-down rituals like having a warm bath, reading quietly or doing some relaxation exercises can all improve your sleep quality and quota.

5 Healthy weight
People with a BMI of 30 or more are considered to be obese, and may experience further heart complications due to this. Dietary changes and increased physical exercise are the two best ways to lose or maintain a healthy weight. See your doctor for help.

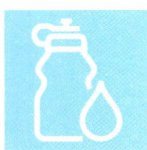

6 Hydration
Staying hydrated helps the heart pump blood more efficiently through the blood vessels. Drinking eight cups of water a day is the recommended option, but sparkling water, unflavoured milk, tea, coffee or a small glass of juice can also assist with hydration. Sugary drinks and alcohol are not recommended.

7 Heart checks
An annual heart health check is essential for monitoring blood pressure, cholesterol, weight and blood glucose levels to identify and address any heart risk factors. They're free for those aged 45 and over, or from age 30 for First Nations peoples. Book in with your GP or local health service.

8 Stress reduction
Meditation, deep breathing, yoga, listening to music, disconnecting from technology or seeing a professional counsellor can all help manage life's daily stressors, which can increase the risk of heart disease.

For more information, visit the Victor Chang Cardiac Research Institute; victorchang.edu.au

The signs of stroke and heart attack

STROKE

- Paralysis, weakness or numbness of the face, arms, legs or on one or both sides of the body
- Facial droop on one or both sides affecting the mouth and/or eyes
- Trouble speaking or understanding, particularly speech that is slurred or garbled
- Loss of vision, sudden blurring or decreased vision in one or both eyes
- Sudden and severe headache
- Vomiting, dizziness or loss of balance
- Difficulty swallowing

HEART ATTACK

- Pain, pressure, discomfort or tightness in the chest, neck, shoulder, jaw, upper back or abdomen
- Shortness of breath with or without chest discomfort
- Pain in one or both arms
- Nausea, vomiting or indigestion
- Hot or cold sweats
- Light-headedness or dizziness
- Unusual feelings of fatigue
- Heart palpitations

RESTART A HEART

A new global initiative urges every person to assist in the event of a cardiac arrest. If you see someone collapse and cease breathing, please follow these steps:

CALL If it is safe to approach, check for a response from the patient and call Triple Zero (000) for instructions.

PUSH If breathing is absent or abnormal, begin CPR. Place the patient on their back, position both hands in the centre of the chest (or two fingers for infants) and compress continually at about one-third depth. Don't be afraid to push hard – you will do more help than harm. Monitor for breathing.

SHOCK If an AED (automated external defibrillator) is available, switch it on and follow the instructions. An AED analyses heart rhythm and may prompt you to shock the patient. Stay clear and continue delivering CPR and following the AED instructions until breathing returns or paramedics arrive.

For more information, visit restartaheart.net

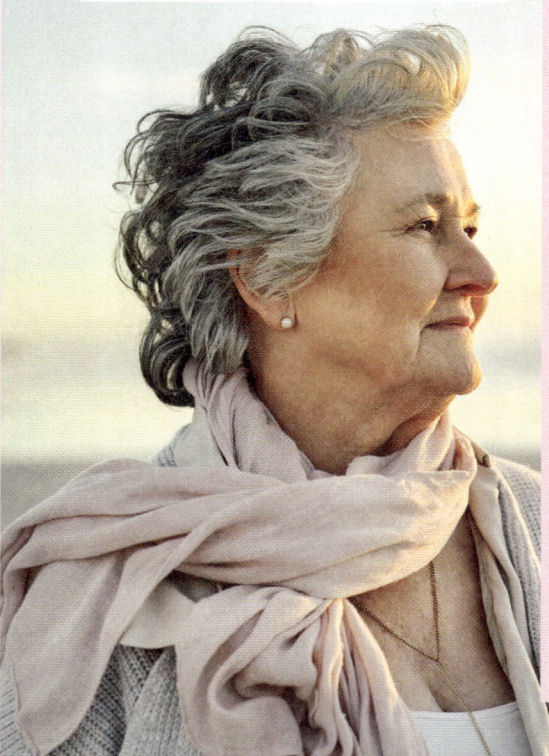

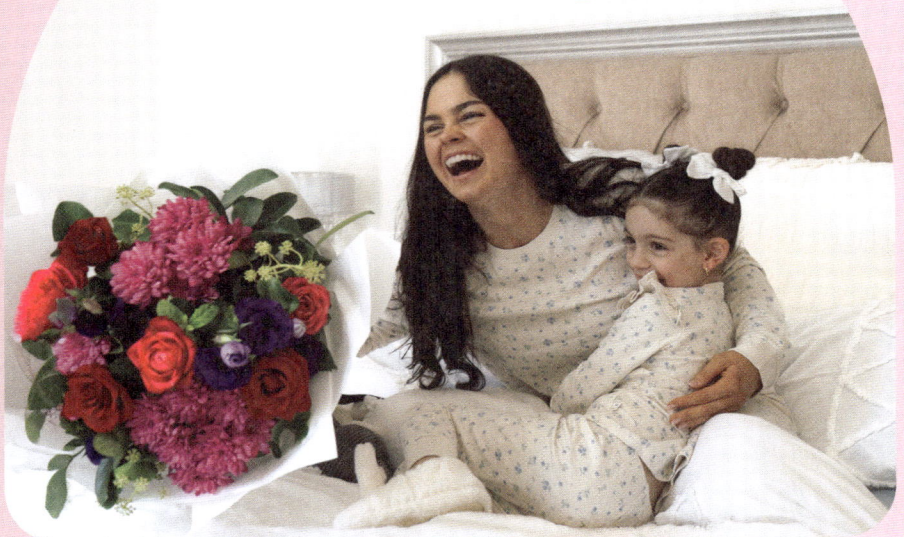

Make every moment brighter

For over 70 years, Australians have turned to Interflora to help express life's most meaningful moments.

From joyful celebrations to heartfelt goodbyes, flowers have always had a way of saying what words often can't.

With a network of more than 500 florists across the country, we're proud to be your local florist—wherever you are. And with same-day delivery available, those important messages never have to wait.

Whether you're sending love across the street or across the world, Interflora makes it easy to stay connected. We deliver to over 145 countries, helping you reach the people who matter most, no matter the distance.

Every bouquet is handcrafted with care and delivered with heart—because at Interflora, we don't just deliver flowers.

We deliver moments to remember.

Get $15 off when you spend $100 at Interflora with code BCT1026*

*Valid until 31/12/26. One use per customer.
Min. spend $100. AUS orders only.
Not valid with other codes.

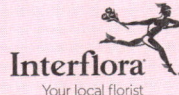

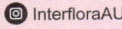 InterfloraAU   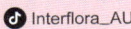 Interflora_AU   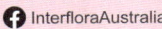 InterfloraAustralia   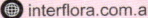 interflora.com.au

	APRIL					
S	M	T	W	T	F	S
			1	2	3	4
5	6	7	8	9	10	11
12	13	14	15	16	17	18
19	20	21	22	23	24	25
26	27	28	29	30		

	MAY					
S	M	T	W	T	F	S
31					1	2
3	4	5	6	7	8	9
10	11	12	13	14	15	16
17	18	19	20	21	22	23
24	25	26	27	28	29	30

	JUNE					
S	M	T	W	T	F	S
	1	2	3	4	5	6
7	8	9	10	11	12	13
14	15	16	17	18	19	20
21	22	23	24	25	26	27
28	29	30				

27 MONDAY

28 TUESDAY

29 WEDNESDAY

30 THURSDAY

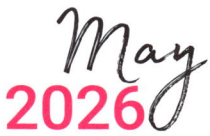

2026

1 FRIDAY

2 SATURDAY

SUPPORT THE 'FOR OUR MUMS' APPEAL ON MAY 7 and have your donation to our breast cancer research doubled! Visit breastcancertrials.org.au.

3 SUNDAY

		APRIL				
S	M	T	W	T	F	S
			1	2	3	4
5	6	7	8	9	10	11
12	13	14	15	16	17	18
19	20	21	22	23	24	25
26	27	28	29	30		

		MAY				
S	M	T	W	T	F	S
31					1	2
3	4	5	6	7	8	9
10	11	12	13	14	15	16
17	18	19	20	21	22	23
24	25	26	27	28	29	30

		JUNE				
S	M	T	W	T	F	S
	1	2	3	4	5	6
7	8	9	10	11	12	13
14	15	16	17	18	19	20
21	22	23	24	25	26	27
28	29	30				

4 MONDAY LABOUR DAY (QLD), MAY DAY (NT)

5 TUESDAY

6 WEDNESDAY

7 THURSDAY

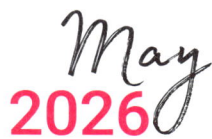
May 2026

8 FRIDAY

9 SATURDAY

CUT DOWN ON SATURATED FATS (butter, fried food, pastries, pies) and ultra-processed foods (sugary breakfast cereals, processed meat, lollies, soft drinks) for optimal heart health.

10 SUNDAY MOTHER'S DAY

		APRIL				
S	M	T	W	T	F	S
			1	2	3	4
5	6	7	8	9	10	11
12	13	14	15	16	17	18
19	20	21	22	23	24	25
26	27	28	29	30		

		MAY				
S	M	T	W	T	F	S
31					1	2
3	4	5	6	7	8	9
10	11	12	13	14	15	16
17	18	19	20	21	22	23
24	25	26	27	28	29	30

		JUNE				
S	M	T	W	T	F	S
	1	2	3	4	5	6
7	8	9	10	11	12	13
14	15	16	17	18	19	20
21	22	23	24	25	26	27
28	29	30				

11 MONDAY

12 TUESDAY

13 WEDNESDAY

14 THURSDAY

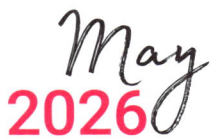
2026

15 FRIDAY

16 SATURDAY

A NUMBER OF PHARMACIES OFFER FREE blood pressure checks and sell or hire out machines to monitor it from home. Visit findapharmacy.com.au to locate options near you.

17 SUNDAY

	APRIL					
S	M	T	W	T	F	S
			1	2	3	4
5	6	7	8	9	10	11
12	13	14	15	16	17	18
19	20	21	22	23	24	25
26	27	28	29	30		

	MAY					
S	M	T	W	T	F	S
31					1	2
3	4	5	6	7	8	9
10	11	12	13	14	15	16
17	18	19	20	21	22	23
24	25	26	27	28	29	30

	JUNE					
S	M	T	W	T	F	S
	1	2	3	4	5	6
7	8	9	10	11	12	13
14	15	16	17	18	19	20
21	22	23	24	25	26	27
28	29	30				

18 MONDAY

19 TUESDAY

20 WEDNESDAY

21 THURSDAY

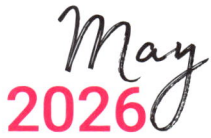
May 2026

22 FRIDAY

23 SATURDAY

WORKING FROM HOME? Set reminders in your calendar to stand up and stretch regularly throughout the day and plan a walk or swim during your lunch break.

24 SUNDAY

	APRIL					
S	M	T	W	T	F	S
			1	2	3	4
5	6	7	8	9	10	11
12	13	14	15	16	17	18
19	20	21	22	23	24	25
26	27	28	29	30		

	MAY					
S	M	T	W	T	F	S
31					1	2
3	4	5	6	7	8	9
10	11	12	13	14	15	16
17	18	19	20	21	22	23
24	25	26	27	28	29	30

	JUNE					
S	M	T	W	T	F	S
	1	2	3	4	5	6
7	8	9	10	11	12	13
14	15	16	17	18	19	20
21	22	23	24	25	26	27
28	29	30				

25 MONDAY

26 TUESDAY NATIONAL SORRY DAY

27 WEDNESDAY EID AL-ADHA (ISLAMIC HOLIDAY)

28 THURSDAY

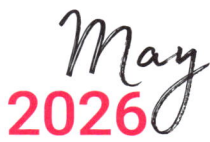
May 2026

29 FRIDAY

30 SATURDAY

ENJOY AT LEAST TWO SERVES OF FISH each week to reduce the risk of heart disease and stroke, lower blood pressure and boost good cholesterol.

31 SUNDAY

WHY I SUPPORT BREAST CANCER TRIALS

My husband, four children and three grandchildren bring joy to my life. I thank God for the strength he gives me every day. My connection with God and faith in him has helped me to stay calm and to believe in the plan he has for my life.

Vainetutai Porio Maka Kea, diagnosed age 57

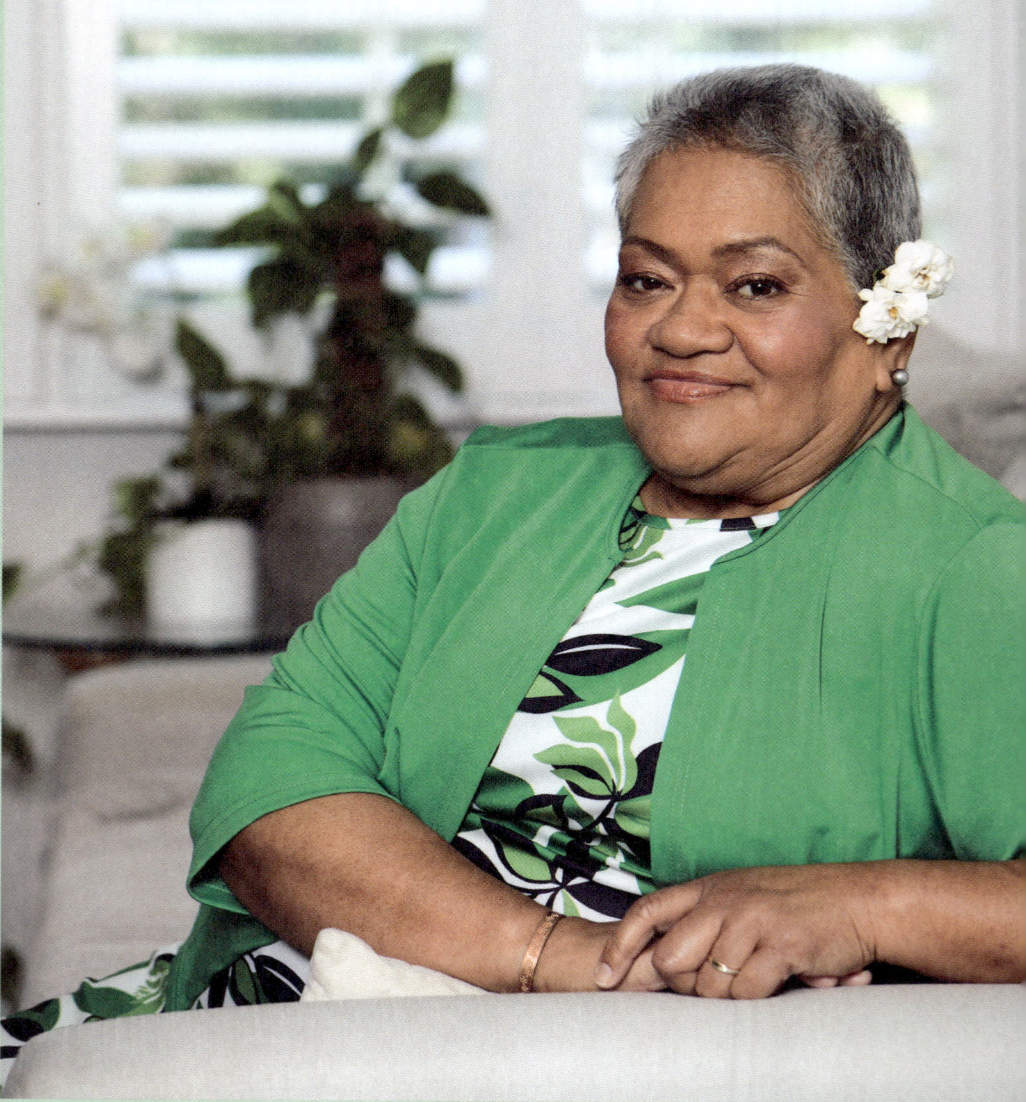

let's talk about
YOUR FINANCES

Your financial position can have a big impact on your emotional, mental and physical wellbeing. Take control of your money to minimise debt, plan for the future and enjoy life along the way.

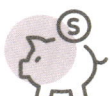

If money matters are a cause of concern, you're not alone. Studies show that 46 per cent of people are dealing with financial worries at least once a week, while 15 per cent are currently in debt. Use the following strategies to regain control of your finances.

REVIEW YOUR CREDIT CARD AND BANK STATEMENTS
This can help you to understand where your money is going and identify ways to cut back your spending on things like unused streaming services, takeaway or luxury items.

ADDRESS DEBT
Take note of any money you owe and prioritise paying off the debt with the highest interest rate first – usually credit cards. If it feels too overwhelming, seek help from the National Debt Helpline; 1800 007 007.

IDENTIFY SPENDING TRIGGERS
Sometimes money problems are the result of unhelpful spending habits or triggers, such as grocery shopping without a list, being lured in by social media ads, impulse buying or spending more due to social pressures. Pinpoint the cues behind your spending and look for ways to address or eliminate them.

PAY ATTENTION TO YOUR SUPER
Compare super funds to find one with a strong long-term performance, low fees, good insurance cover and member benefits. Consolidate super accounts into one to avoid additional fees and if possible, make extra contributions to top it up.

BE SCAM-SAVVY
Scams are everywhere, costing Australians billions of dollars each year. Avoid falling victim by following these steps: stop and ask yourself if the email or phone call seems legitimate; never click unfamiliar links or provide personal details over the phone or email; if in doubt contact the bank or organisation to check.

LEARN MORE ABOUT MONEY
Be confident managing your finances by arming yourself with information. Read articles, listen to podcasts, subscribe to newsletters, take an online course or seek advice from a financial planner.

> *Put together a monthly budget to map out the money you have and help plan for upcoming bills and other expenses.*

The financial impact of career breaks

It's an unfortunate fact that for many women, taking a break from their careers to raise children can leave them more financially worse off than their partners. Taking leave or working reduced hours to study, travel or care for a family member can also lead to financial strain. Read on to discover the pitfalls and potential solutions.

EARNING CAPACITY

Reducing your hours or taking extended leave can put a dent in your income, so consider ways to manage your financial responsibilities during this time. Can you dip into your savings? Are you eligible for assistance schemes like Parental Leave Pay or Carer's Allowance? Also look for ways to reduce spending or bring in extra income while not working.

EXTRA EXPENSES

There may be costs associated with your change in circumstance. For example, if you're on maternity leave, there will be items needed for the baby and possibly childcare fees if you return to work. If you're studying, you may need to purchase textbooks or a laptop. Where possible, look into discounts, rebates and special deals and source good quality baby items and textbooks second-hand.

MORTGAGE OR RENTAL STRESS

Government-funded parental leave payments are based on the minimum wage, so your household income may be impacted. This in turn can make it difficult to meet your rent or mortgage payments. As a first step, call your bank to ask about financial hardship assistance or speak to your landlord or rental agent. You may be able to negotiate a temporary halt on repayments or a payment plan, or in the case of your mortgage, switch to interest-only payments or refinance your loan.

SUPERANNUATION

You generally won't earn super if you're taking long periods of unpaid leave and you may also see an impact if you reduce your hours for an extended period. Look into making a personal after-tax contribution or whether your spouse can make a spouse contribution on your behalf. There may be tax benefits for both.

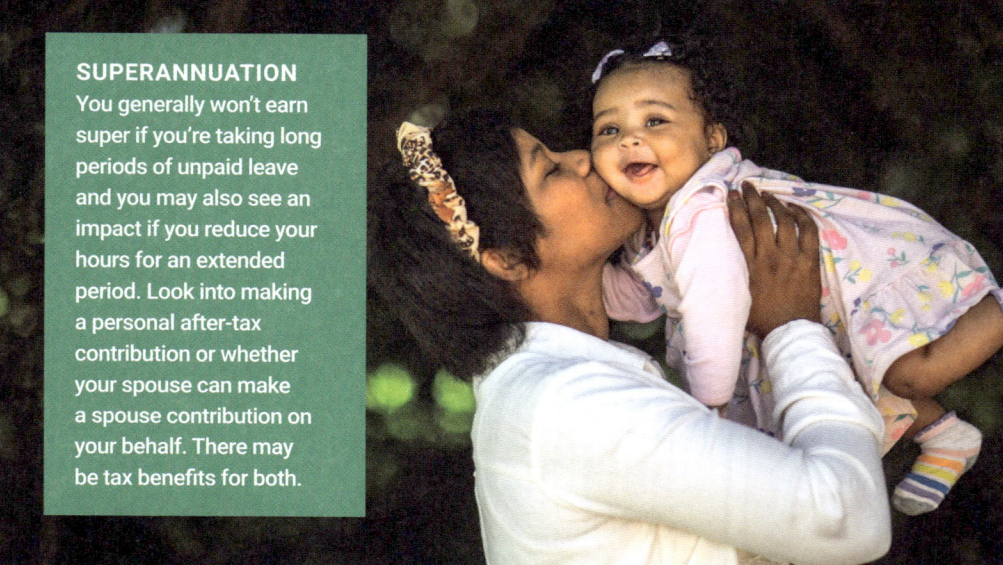

Will-writing tips for every age

While some Australians may think having a will is an unnecessary step or something that can be left until later in life, the truth is that everyone over the age of 18 should have one. More than just a piece of paper, a will is a plan for the future, ensuring that your wishes are met and your assets are managed the way you want, sparing your loved ones additional stress. Here's what to consider at various stages of life.

YOUNG ADULTS

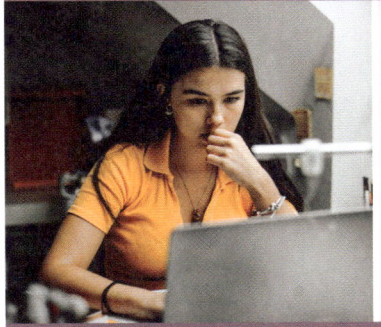

At this age, your assets might include bank accounts, a car or personal items of value. Think who you would like to receive these assets in the event of your death, and if you have a pet, who will care for it. Also consider any liabilities, such as credit card debt, student debt or personal loans, which will be paid from your assets. Elect a responsible person to handle the execution of your estate – a family member, trusted friend or an independent trustee organisation or solicitor. Also make sure you have nominated a beneficiary on your super account.

PARENTS

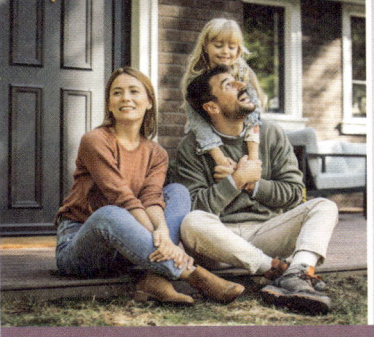

Update your will to reflect any changes in your life situation – for example if you get married or divorced, have children or your financial assets change. Nominate someone to care for young children if both parents pass away. You may also want to set up a testamentary trust, to hold your assets until children come of age. Keep relevant documents in one place and leave details of where to find them – things like your birth certificate, marriage certificate, life insurance, medical insurance, house deeds, bank account details and superannuation papers.

RETIREES

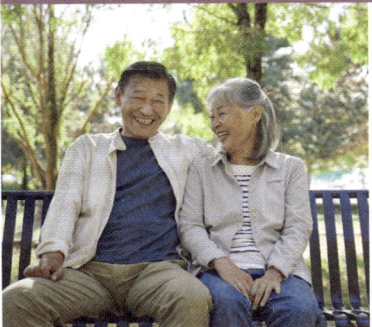

Make sure your will is up to date and if you haven't already, consider appointing an Enduring Power of Attorney (to make financial and legal decisions) and an Enduring Guardianship (for personal, lifestyle and medical decisions). Both can act on your behalf if you're unable to yourself. An advanced healthcare directive outlines what treatments you would like to receive or refuse in the event of an incapacitating illness or injury. You may also like to outline your funeral arrangements or prepay for your funeral – leave a copy of this information with your executor.

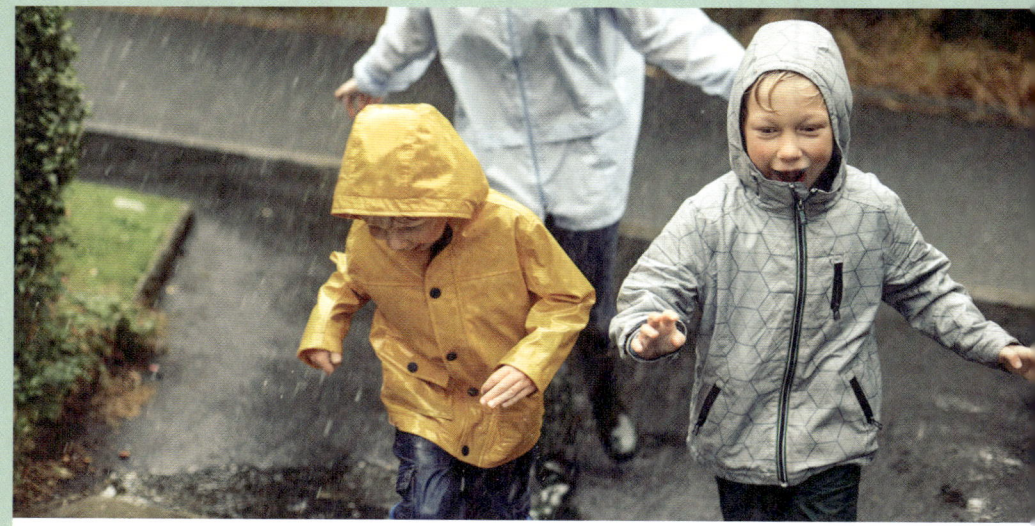

The importance of a rainy-day fund

Whether you're comfortably living within your means or struggling to make ends meet, unexpected life events can put a strain on your finances. Job loss, urgent repairs, pet care, medical procedures, surprise bills, unplanned travel or funeral expenses are just some of the costs that we don't always plan for, and it can be disheartening having to dip into your savings or max out your credit card to cover them. That's where a rainy-day fund comes in.

WHAT IS A RAINY-DAY FUND?
Also known as an emergency fund, this is a separate account or sum of money earmarked for emergencies. A rainy-day fund should be kept separate to savings and shouldn't be a replacement for insurance (although you may like to use it for out of pocket expenses that insurance policies or Medicare won't cover).

HOW MUCH SHOULD YOU HAVE IN A RAINY-DAY FUND?
The amount you need will depend on your personal circumstances. If you're single or renting you may need less than someone with a mortgage or dependents. Think about the things in your life that you can't do without – for example, your income, your car, your refrigerator or a beloved pet – and what is a reasonable amount that would cover any costs if something went wrong? As a general rule, try to save enough for three-to-six months' worth of expenses. If this is not realistic, aim for an amount like $1000 (around $20 per week) and add to it when you can.

HOW TO GET STARTED
Use the Budget Planner at the front of this diary to track your income and expenses and look for areas where you can potentially save. Use a new or existing account to keep your rainy-day savings separate to everyday spending money. A high-interest savings or offset account is good, but avoid term deposits, which can't always be accessed when you need the funds. Set up a recurring transfer into this rainy-day account so you don't have to think about it. Don't hesitate to use this money when emergencies arise – you can always build it up again at a later date.

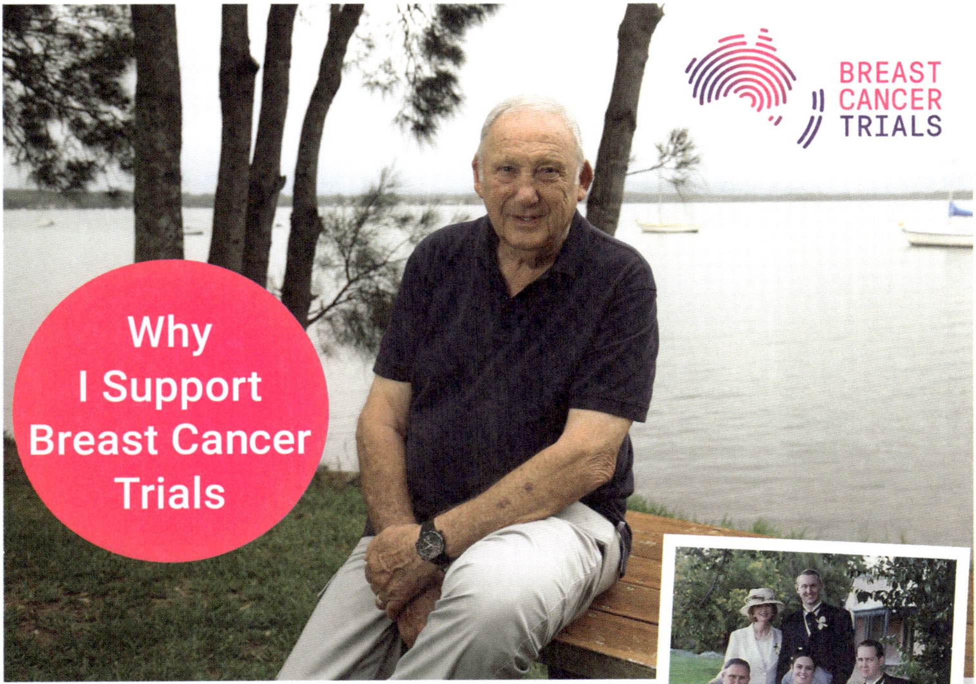

BREAST CANCER TRIALS

Why I Support Breast Cancer Trials

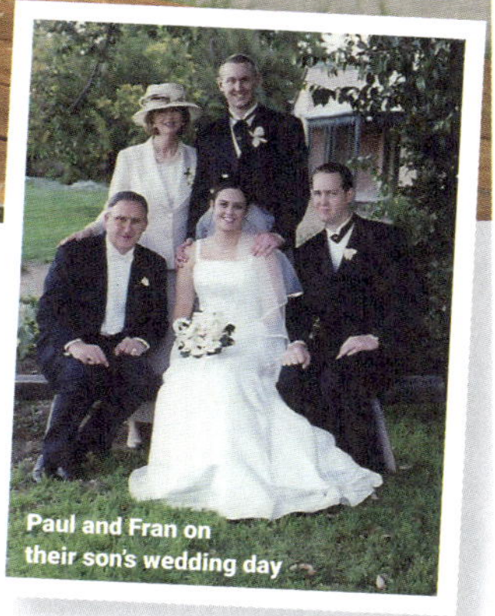

Paul and Fran on their son's wedding day

My late wife Fran and I had a wonderful life together with our sons, but it came to an end when she passed away from breast cancer at age 60.

When anyone goes through this or watches their cherished loved one go through it and see your family and its dreams for the future destroyed, you just can't say 'why us?' and do nothing about it.

I have chosen to leave a gift in my will to Breast Cancer Trials because I'm convinced that well-funded research will find solutions so that no more women of any age will suffer the indignities and pain of breast cancer, and the devastation it causes families like mine will stop.

No one fought harder than my late wife, and I'm not going to stop fighting because she never gave up and I'm not going to either.

CREATE A LASTING LEGACY BY INCLUDING BREAST CANCER TRIALS IN YOUR WILL TODAY.

For more information please contact 1800 423 444, bequestenquiries@bctrials.org.au, scan this QR code or visit www.breastcancertrials.org.au/gifts-in-wills

		MAY				
S	M	T	W	T	F	S
31					1	2
3	4	5	6	7	8	9
10	11	12	13	14	15	16
17	18	19	20	21	22	23
24	25	26	27	28	29	30

		JUNE				
S	M	T	W	T	F	S
	1	2	3	4	5	6
7	8	9	10	11	12	13
14	15	16	17	18	19	20
21	22	23	24	25	26	27
28	29	30				

		JULY				
S	M	T	W	T	F	S
			1	2	3	4
5	6	7	8	9	10	11
12	13	14	15	16	17	18
19	20	21	22	23	24	25
26	27	28	29	30	31	

1 MONDAY WESTERN AUSTRALIA DAY (WA), RECONCILIATION DAY (ACT)

2 TUESDAY

3 WEDNESDAY

4 THURSDAY

June
2026

5 FRIDAY

6 SATURDAY

> **REVIEW YOUR INSURANCE POLICIES** every year to ensure they're offering you the best deal and providing adequate coverage for your needs.

7 SUNDAY

	M	A Y				
S	M	T	W	T	F	S
31					1	2
3	4	5	6	7	8	9
10	11	12	13	14	15	16
17	18	19	20	21	22	23
24	25	26	27	28	29	30

		J U N E				
S	M	T	W	T	F	S
	1	2	3	4	5	6
7	8	9	10	11	12	13
14	15	16	17	18	19	20
21	22	23	24	25	26	27
28	29	30				

		J U L Y				
S	M	T	W	T	F	S
			1	2	3	4
5	6	7	8	9	10	11
12	13	14	15	16	17	18
19	20	21	22	23	24	25
26	27	28	29	30	31	

8 MONDAY KING'S BIRTHDAY (ACT, NSW, NT, SA, TAS, VIC)

9 TUESDAY

10 WEDNESDAY

11 THURSDAY

June
2026

12 FRIDAY

13 SATURDAY

> **AVOID TAKING OUT A HIGH-INTEREST LOAN** to cover an unexpected bill. Instead, consider asking your service provider for an interest-free payment plan.

14 SUNDAY

	MAY					
S	M	T	W	T	F	S
31					1	2
3	4	5	6	7	8	9
10	11	12	13	14	15	16
17	18	19	20	21	22	23
24	25	26	27	28	29	30

	JUNE					
S	M	T	W	T	F	S
	1	2	3	4	5	6
7	8	9	10	11	12	13
14	15	16	17	18	19	20
21	22	23	24	25	26	27
28	29	30				

	JULY					
S	M	T	W	T	F	S
			1	2	3	4
5	6	7	8	9	10	11
12	13	14	15	16	17	18
19	20	21	22	23	24	25
26	27	28	29	30	31	

15 MONDAY

16 TUESDAY

17 WEDNESDAY MUHARRAM/ISLAMIC NEW YEAR

18 THURSDAY

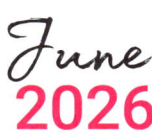
June
2026

19 FRIDAY

20 SATURDAY

PLEASE MAKE A DONATION

to breast cancer research by June 30. You can claim it as a tax deduction in your tax return. Call 1800 423 444 or visit breastcancertrials.org.au.

21 SUNDAY

		MAY				
S	M	T	W	T	F	S
31					1	2
3	4	5	6	7	8	9
10	11	12	13	14	15	16
17	18	19	20	21	22	23
24	25	26	27	28	29	30

		JUNE				
S	M	T	W	T	F	S
	1	2	3	4	5	6
7	8	9	10	11	12	13
14	15	16	17	18	19	20
21	22	23	24	25	26	27
28	29	30				

		JULY				
S	M	T	W	T	F	S
			1	2	3	4
5	6	7	8	9	10	11
12	13	14	15	16	17	18
19	20	21	22	23	24	25
26	27	28	29	30	31	

22 MONDAY

23 TUESDAY

24 WEDNESDAY

25 THURSDAY

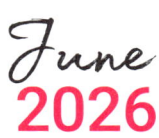
June
2026

26 FRIDAY

27 SATURDAY

> **PROTECT YOURSELF FROM FRAUD**
> by regularly changing passwords, using two-factor authentication and checking for scam alerts from government sources.

28 SUNDAY

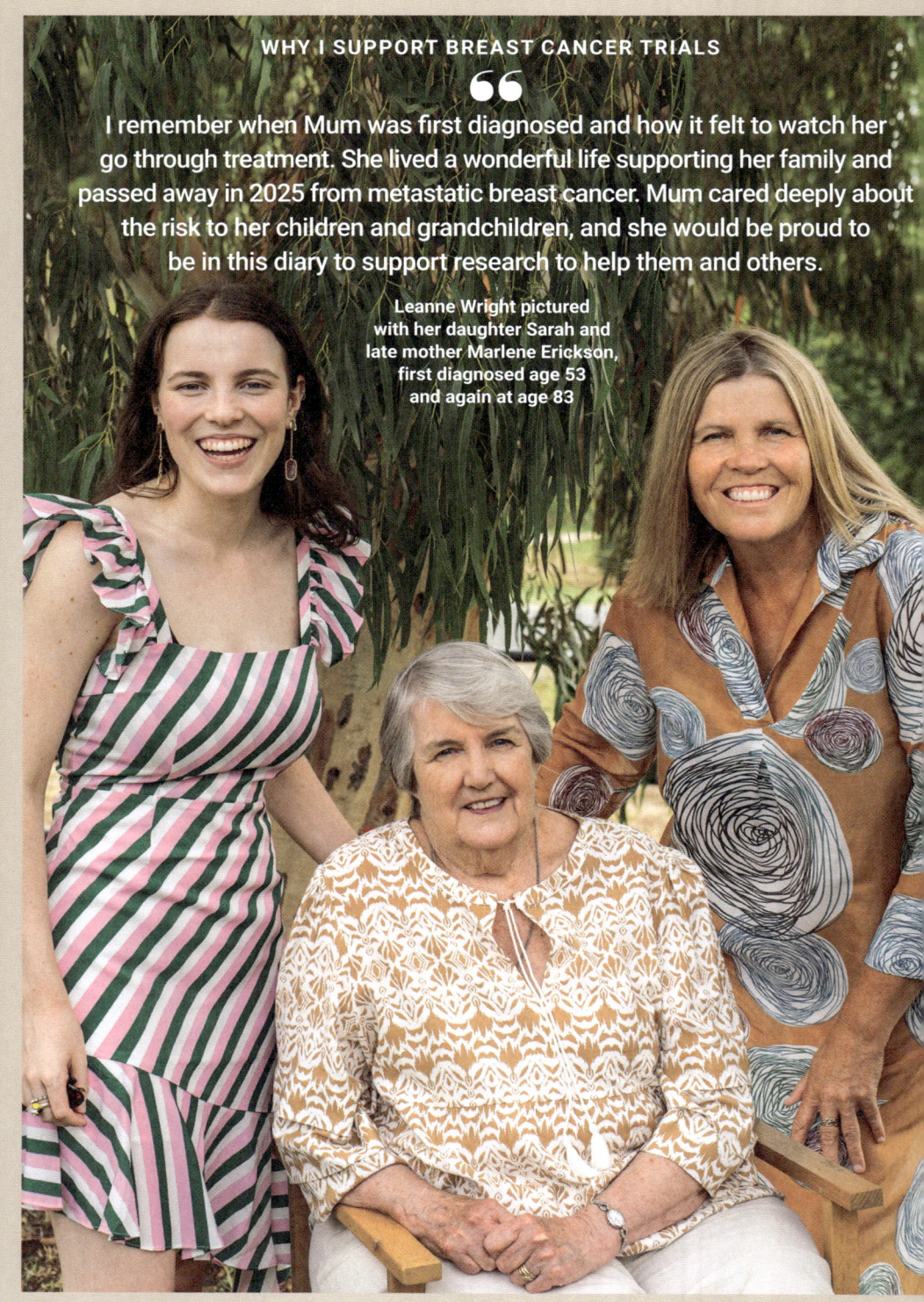

let's talk about
AGEING

Australians are living longer, with an average life expectancy of 83 years. Get the most from your later years by adopting healthy habits, fostering relationships and developing a positive outlook.

Body image issues can affect people of all ages, genders and backgrounds. While it often occurs in late childhood and adolescence, body dissatisfaction can continue into midlife, when fluctuating hormones, weight shifts and the signs of ageing bring a whole new dimension. Rather than resorting to harsh diets or strict exercise regimes, try these strategies to view your body in a more positive light.

5 WAYS TO BOOST BODY CONFIDENCE AFTER AGE 40

1 Reframe your mindset
Take note of your inner monologue around your body and its appearance and practise turning negative self-talk into positive self-talk. Appreciate that every body is unique and focus on all the incredible things that your body is capable of, such as running a marathon, giving birth or simply keeping you alive. Acknowledge that getting older is a good thing and not to be taken for granted.

2 Edit your social media
Every day we're exposed to unrealistic body ideals in the form of stylised images and ads targeting weight loss or fad diets. Control your exposure by following people and accounts that make you feel good, seeking out older role models and understanding the intent behind the posts.

3 Dress for you
Remember this: clothes should fit you; you don't need to change to fit them. Sort through your wardrobe and donate or recycle any items that feel uncomfortable, then shop for affordable replacements, choosing styles and colours that help you look and feel good.

4 Exercise for fun
When exercise feels like a chore or an obligation, it's not enjoyable. Remove the pressure and find an activity that you love. Short bursts of activity can also be beneficial, so spread it across the day and enjoy the endorphin release.

5 Ask for help
If you find you're obsessively thinking about your body, comparing your appearance to others', frequently weighing or checking yourself in the mirror or withdrawing from loved ones and things you enjoy, speak to your GP or a counsellor.

For more information, visit the Butterfly Foundation; butterfly.org.au

Spotlight on dementia

Dementia is the term used to describe a group of conditions that cause a progressive decline in a person's cognitive function. There are many forms of dementia, the most common being Alzheimer's disease. In 2025, there were an estimated 433,300 Australians living with dementia, including 29,000 people under the age of 65, and it was the leading cause of death for women. Without significant intervention, the number of people in Australian with dementia is expected to increase to an estimated 812,500 by 2054.

CAUSES
For many people, the exact cause of their dementia is not known, however, family history can play a part. We also know that 45 per cent of cases might be avoided by focusing on modifiable factors – obesity, smoking, high blood pressure, hearing loss, depression and diabetes can all increase the risk.

SYMPTOMS
The experience of dementia varies from person to person, with some days better than others. Symptoms may include:
- **Memory decline** Difficulty recalling recent events, names or people, not recognising family and friends, forgetting how to dress or bathe.
- **Impaired thinking** Confusion, trouble concentrating, reasoning or problem solving, struggling to complete everyday tasks, inability to judge distances, directions or time, mixing up words or repeating yourself.
- **Altered mood** Feeling less motivated, social apathy and withdrawal, more prone to depression, anxiety and agitation, not yourself.
- **Changes in behaviour** Disturbed sleep, becoming restless, wandering, saying or doing things that are out of character, rapid mood swings.

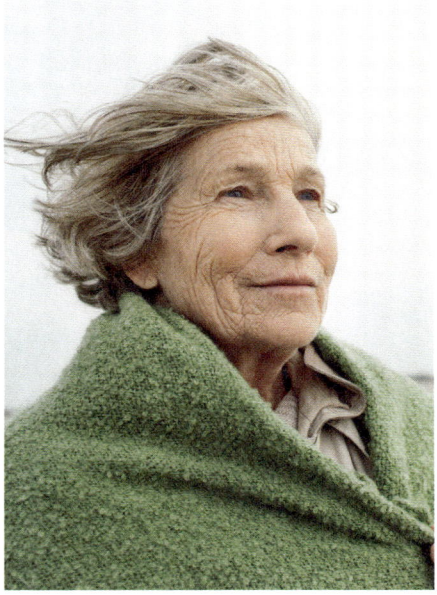

DIAGNOSIS AND TREATMENT While there is no single conclusive test to diagnose dementia, and no cure, your GP or specialist can do a combination of cognitive and medical assessments to make a diagnosis. Some medications may help with dementia symptoms and you can also focus on maintaining brain health with regular exercise, social interactions and mental stimulation from word or maths puzzles.

For more information, visit Dementia Australia; dementia.org.au

Cooking for one

When you're preparing meals for just yourself, it can start to feel like a bit of a chore. Follow these tips to make it work for you.

SHOP SMART
Plan out your meals before you go grocery shopping, using the same ingredients to reduce waste. Stock up on staples with a longer shelf life, like canned legumes and beans, tinned tomatoes, pasta, rice, noodles, canned fruit, dried herbs and spices and frozen vegetables. Single-use items or smaller quantities can work out to be more expensive, so buy in bulk and portion into single serves at home.

MAKE IT A FUN CHALLENGE
Take the monotony out of cooking for one by giving yourself a challenge. It might be trying one new recipe or ingredient each week, plating up your food in fancy ways, thinking up creative ideas to use leftovers or growing your own produce to cook with.

EMBRACE "BRINNER"
There's something about eating breakfast at dinner time that feels a little indulgent, and many breakfast options tick off a host of nutritional needs. Try eggs or baked beans on wholegrain toast, porridge topped with nuts or pancakes with fruit and yoghurt.

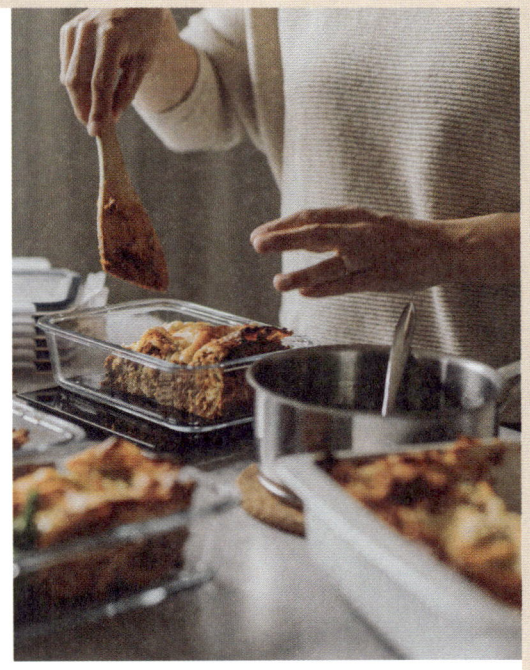

COOK ONCE, EAT FOR DAYS
Batch-cook meals like casseroles, soups, bolognese, meatballs, dumplings and curries and portion into single serves. Enjoy for lunch or dinner or keep in the freezer to have a range of options on hand.

GET THE RIGHT BALANCE
Follow the plate model to ensure you're eating a balanced meal: half a plate of fruit, vegetables or salad, a quarter of the plate for lean protein and the other quarter for grains and cereals. Also consult the table below.

Recommended daily serves for women	Vegetables and legumes	Fruit	Grains	Lean meat, fish, poultry, eggs, nuts, seeds	Milk, yoghurt, cheese and alternatives
19-50 years	5	2	6	2.5	2.5
51-70 years	5	2	4	2	4
70 years+	5	2	3	2	4
Pregnant	5	2	8.5	3.5	2.5
Breastfeeding	7.5	2	9	2.5	2.5

Caring for older parents

With Australians living longer and sometimes delaying having children, many people in their 40s and 50s are now juggling the needs of their own family with those of their ageing parent(s). This role reversal – where the child now cares for their parent – can be challenging for both parties. The older parents may grapple with loss of independence, declining health and changes in their living circumstances, while the adult children may experience increased stress, fatigue, financial implications and the sad reminder of their parents' mortality. Try these steps to make this journey a little easier, approaching each day with empathy and respect.

ESTABLISH BOUNDARIES
Navigate this shift in your relationship by setting some mutually beneficial boundaries. This might include having set times or days when you visit each other, choosing doctors or specialists in a location that is convenient for you both or delegating tasks like meal or grocery delivery to outside providers.

SEEK LEGAL ADVICE
Your parents' ability to make decisions may change as they age. Suggest they see a solicitor to establish an Enduring Power of Attorney to make legal and financial decisions or Enduring Guardianship for health, medical and lifestyle decisions. The person(s) appointed can act on your parents' behalf if they're unable to.

DON'T DO IT ALONE
Reach out to siblings, family members and support agencies like Carers Australia for help with your parents' care. Seek counselling or support as needed. And encourage your parents to pursue friendships and activities.

TALK NOW ABOUT THE FUTURE
Start an open conversation with your parents about how they would like to spend the rest of their life, discussing living arrangements, financial responsibilities, health needs and household tasks. Explore government assistance options through My Aged Care, and have an emergency healthcare plan in place should any medical needs arise down the track.

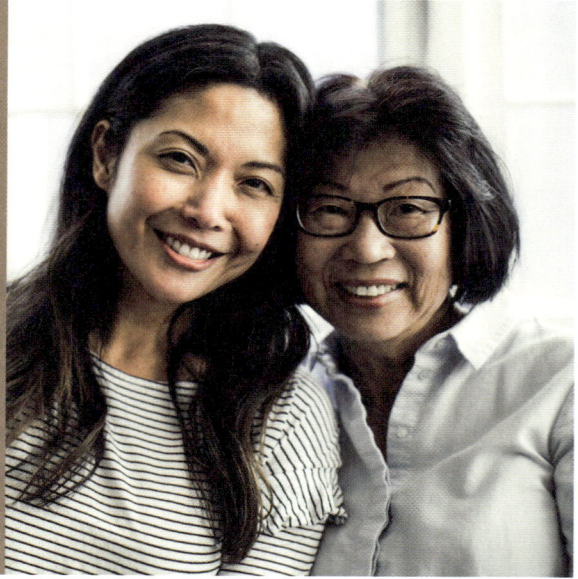

For more information, visit Carers Australia; carersaustralia.com.au

Home safety tips

As you get older, creating a safe environment is important for staying at home for longer and reducing the risk of falls. Take the time making some changes around your home now to help eliminate any potential hazards and guard against accidents.

Have good lighting, especially motion-activated lights near stairs and between the bed and bathroom.

Make sure your home has a working smoke alarm and a fire blanket or fire extinguisher within easy reach.

Install grab rails in the bathroom and support rails near any steps.

Choose sturdy chairs and beds that are easy to get out of and tables and benches without sharp corners.

Install a ramp to your front door or handrails at the front steps.

Keep hallways and walkways clear of clutter.

Use adhesive strips on all rugs and mats and replace or repair worn areas, long threads and holes in carpet.

Clear leaves, moss and lichen from outdoor paths, as they can become slippery to walk on when wet.

Repair cracked, broken or uneven pathway pavers; refer public footpaths to your local council.

Mark the edge of steps with white paint for easy visibility and keep them well lit at night.

Avoid using ladders – ask for assistance if you need to access something out of reach.

		JUNE				
S	M	T	W	T	F	S
	1	2	3	4	5	6
7	8	9	10	11	12	13
14	15	16	17	18	19	20
21	22	23	24	25	26	27
28	29	30				

		JULY				
S	M	T	W	T	F	S
			1	2	3	4
5	6	7	8	9	10	11
12	13	14	15	16	17	18
19	20	21	22	23	24	25
26	27	28	29	30	31	

		AUGUST				
S	M	T	W	T	F	S
30	31					1
2	3	4	5	6	7	8
9	10	11	12	13	14	15
16	17	18	19	20	21	22
23	24	25	26	27	28	29

29 MONDAY

30 TUESDAY

1 WEDNESDAY

2 THURSDAY

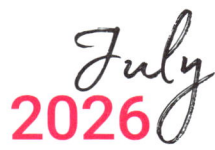
July 2026

3 FRIDAY

4 SATURDAY

CONCERNED ABOUT CHANGES IN YOUR MEMORY? Try the free BrainTrack app by Dementia Australia to test your cognition and share the data with your GP.

5 SUNDAY NAIDOC WEEK BEGINS

		JUNE				
S	M	T	W	T	F	S
	1	2	3	4	5	6
7	8	9	10	11	12	13
14	15	16	17	18	19	20
21	22	23	24	25	26	27
28	29	30				

		JULY				
S	M	T	W	T	F	S
			1	2	3	4
5	6	7	8	9	10	11
12	13	14	15	16	17	18
19	20	21	22	23	24	25
26	27	28	29	30	31	

		AUGUST				
S	M	T	W	T	F	S
30	31					1
2	3	4	5	6	7	8
9	10	11	12	13	14	15
16	17	18	19	20	21	22
23	24	25	26	27	28	29

6 MONDAY

7 TUESDAY

8 WEDNESDAY

9 THURSDAY

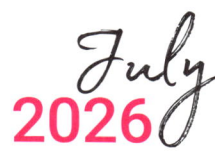
July 2026

10 FRIDAY

11 SATURDAY

THE RISK OF DEVELOPING SHINGLES increases with age and for those with weakened immune systems. Reduce your risk and get vaccinated – it's free from age 65.

12 SUNDAY

		JUNE				
S	M	T	W	T	F	S
	1	2	3	4	5	6
7	8	9	10	11	12	13
14	15	16	17	18	19	20
21	22	23	24	25	26	27
28	29	30				

		JULY				
S	M	T	W	T	F	S
			1	2	3	4
5	6	7	8	9	10	11
12	13	14	15	16	17	18
19	20	21	22	23	24	25
26	27	28	29	30	31	

		AUGUST				
S	M	T	W	T	F	S
30	31					1
2	3	4	5	6	7	8
9	10	11	12	13	14	15
16	17	18	19	20	21	22
23	24	25	26	27	28	29

13 MONDAY

14 TUESDAY BASTILLE DAY (FRANCE)

15 WEDNESDAY

16 THURSDAY

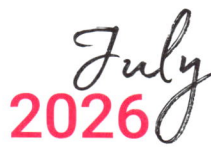
July 2026

17 FRIDAY

18 SATURDAY

HAVE YOUR EYES TESTED EVERY YEAR after age 65 to reduce your risk of falls, and visit your podiatrist regularly to minimise foot problems and to stay mobile.

19 SUNDAY

		JUNE				
S	M	T	W	T	F	S
	1	2	3	4	5	6
7	8	9	10	11	12	13
14	15	16	17	18	19	20
21	22	23	24	25	26	27
28	29	30				

		JULY				
S	M	T	W	T	F	S
			1	2	3	4
5	6	7	8	9	10	11
12	13	14	15	16	17	18
19	20	21	22	23	24	25
26	27	28	29	30	31	

		AUGUST				
S	M	T	W	T	F	S
30	31					1
2	3	4	5	6	7	8
9	10	11	12	13	14	15
16	17	18	19	20	21	22
23	24	25	26	27	28	29

20 MONDAY

21 TUESDAY

22 WEDNESDAY

23 THURSDAY

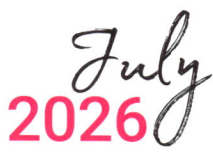

July 2026

24 FRIDAY

25 SATURDAY

BOOK A HOLIDAY!
Studies show that having new experiences and meeting new people can help maintain cognitive and mental health.

26 SUNDAY

	JUNE					
S	M	T	W	T	F	S
	1	2	3	4	5	6
7	8	9	10	11	12	13
14	15	16	17	18	19	20
21	22	23	24	25	26	27
28	29	30				

	JULY					
S	M	T	W	T	F	S
			1	2	3	4
5	6	7	8	9	10	11
12	13	14	15	16	17	18
19	20	21	22	23	24	25
26	27	28	29	30	31	

	AUGUST					
S	M	T	W	T	F	S
30	31					1
2	3	4	5	6	7	8
9	10	11	12	13	14	15
16	17	18	19	20	21	22
23	24	25	26	27	28	29

27 MONDAY

28 TUESDAY

29 WEDNESDAY

30 THURSDAY

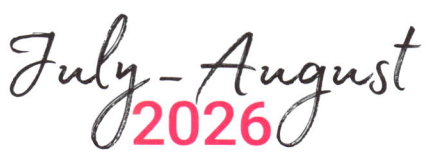

July – August 2026

31 FRIDAY

1 SATURDAY

IF YOU LIVE ALONE OR DON'T DRIVE, utilise community transport and ride-share services to continue attending social events and appointments.

2 SUNDAY

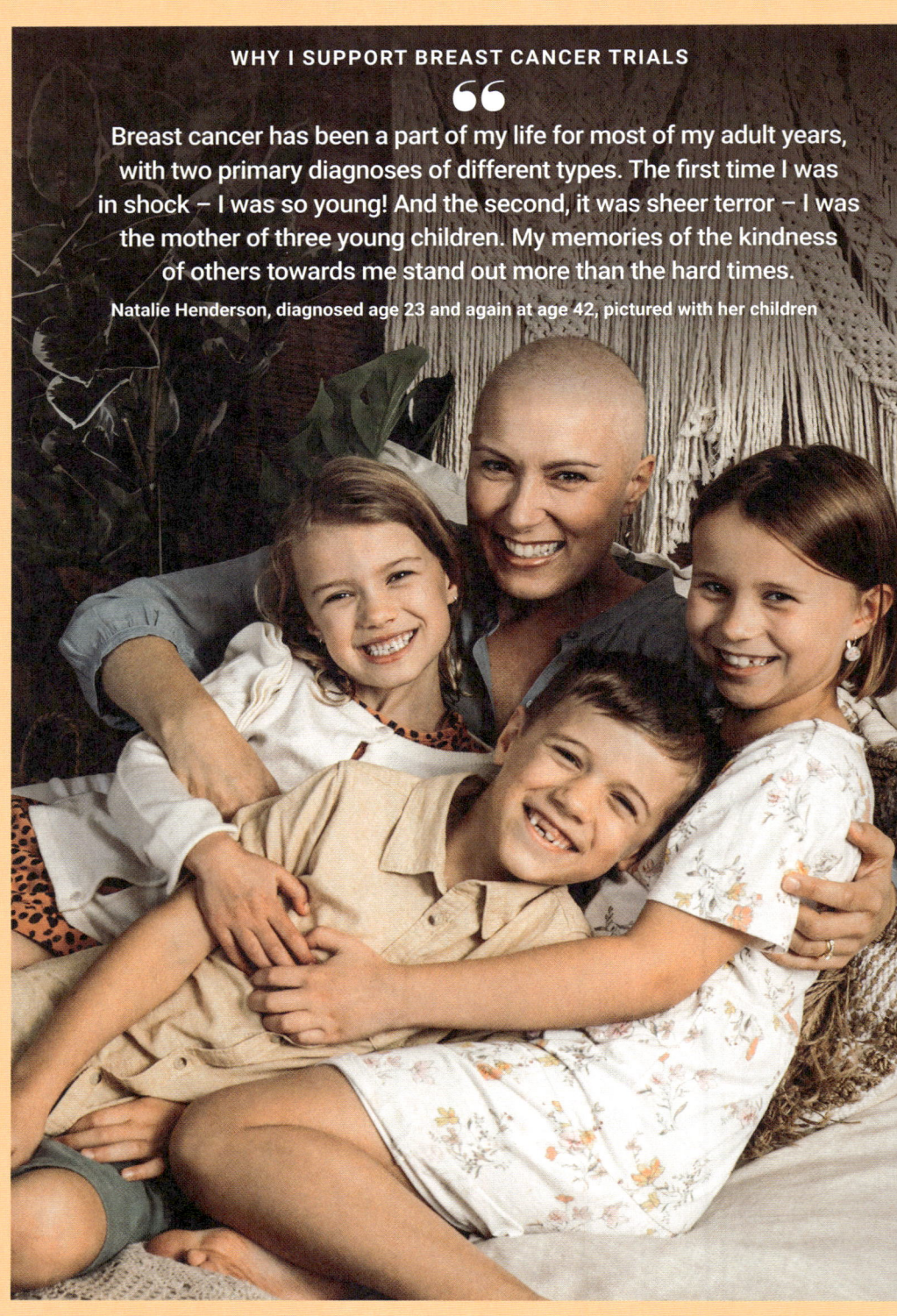

WHY I SUPPORT BREAST CANCER TRIALS

❝ Breast cancer has been a part of my life for most of my adult years, with two primary diagnoses of different types. The first time I was in shock – I was so young! And the second, it was sheer terror – I was the mother of three young children. My memories of the kindness of others towards me stand out more than the hard times.

Natalie Henderson, diagnosed age 23 and again at age 42, pictured with her children

let's talk about
FAMILY

Caring for a family can be both rewarding and challenging. Read on for helpful advice on navigating technology, catering for varying nutritional needs and nurturing these important relationships.

Illnesses like cold viruses and tummy bugs can spread easily among families, which may be cause for frustration or distress. You can often care for family members at home by giving them lots of fluids to avoid dehydration, administering paracetamol or ibuprofen for fever or pain and encouraging plenty of rest. If symptoms persist or worsen, seek medical help. The checklist below is a useful guide.

FEELING UNWELL AND NOT SURE WHAT TO DO NEXT?

Treat at home and ask a pharmacist about over-the-counter medical options for the following symptoms...
- Headache, sore throat or fever
- Blocked/runny nose, sneezing, coughing
- Mild bites, stings and skin rashes
- Vomiting or diarrhoea
- Low energy or appetite.

See your GP if the patient...
- Has had a fever, vomiting or diarrhoea for more than two days
- Is passing less urine than usual
- Isn't drinking well
- Isn't responding to over-the-counter medications
- Develops a lump or swelling
- Symptoms persist or worsen.

Attend your nearest emergency department or call Triple Zero (000) if the patient...
- Becomes unwell very quickly
- Collapses suddenly
- Experiences chest pain
- Has uncontrollable bleeding
- Is under 3 months old and has a fever
- Seems very drowsy, won't wake easily or becomes floppy when you pick them up
- Experiences seizures
- Displays changes in their breathing
- Has a purplish, red or bluish rash
- Complains of a severe headache
- Has difficulty looking at light
- Vomits frequently or is vomiting green fluid or blood
- Has pain that doesn't go away with medicine.

How to help your family avoid getting sick
- Make sure vaccinations are up to date, including annual influenza vaccinations.
- Teach them good hygiene practices, such as washing hands well with soap, not sharing food or drink bottles and coughing into their elbows.
- Ensure they get enough sleep.
- Serve them a balanced diet.

For more information, visit Healthdirect; healthdirect.gov.au

7 ways to connect with your grandchildren

Being a grandparent can be incredibly rewarding and offers benefits for all involved. Spending time with young people can slow cognitive decline and the onset of dementia in older generations, as well as helping to maintain physical fitness. Grandkids benefit from improved emotional connection, growth and learning, while their parents receive additional support and time for self-care. Make the most of this special relationship with these suggestions.

1 Find shared interests To foster a deeper connection, learn about your grandchild's favourite activities, TV shows, hobbies or sports or ask them to tell you about their favourite subject at school.

2 Embrace technology Today's kids are well versed in digital technology, so find ways to connect via video calls, text messages or group chats (particularly useful if you live far apart or are travelling). You might learn a few new skills in the process.

3 Share stories and memories Teach them about their family history by sharing stories and photos from your childhood and handing down family heirlooms or recipes.

4 Attend events Be there for your grandchildren at all their important milestones, such as birthdays, performances, sporting games and award presentations.

5 Create traditions Give them something to look forward to by adding regularity to your catch-ups. It might be a phone call at the same time each week, enjoying a meal at a favourite place or shared holiday traditions.

6 Teach them something new Lean on your years of experience and knowledge to expose grandchildren to new interests, skills and perspectives. For instance, teach them how to play an instrument, a second language or how to change a tyre.

7 Plan memorable activities Make your time together count by planning some fun experiences or outings that they will look back on later in life. Simple is often best – try baking, fishing, playing board games, gardening or taking a holiday together.

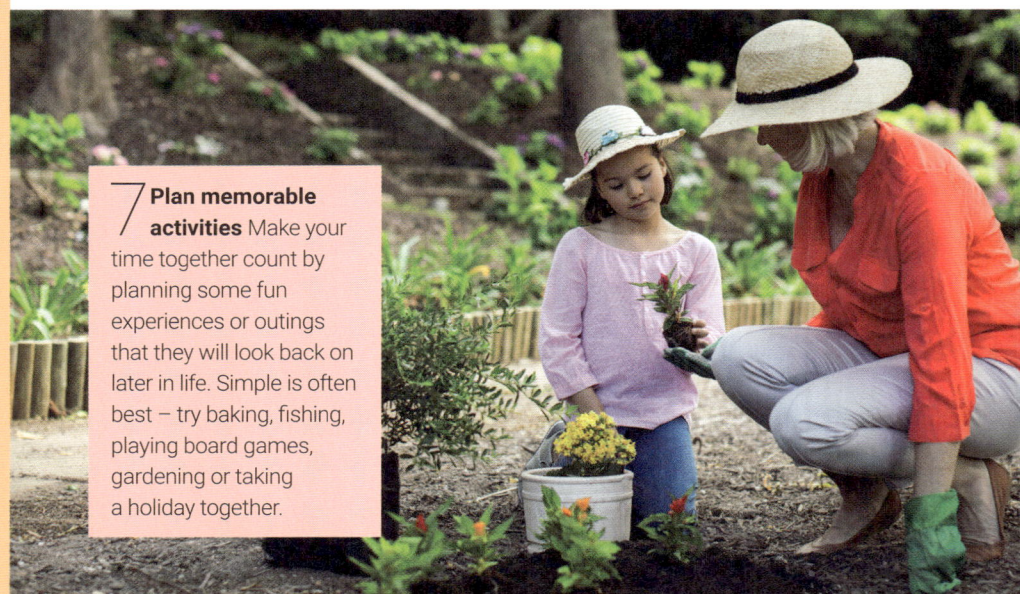

Calcium-rich family meal ideas

Recent surveys indicate that over half of all Australians aged two years and over don't consume enough calcium. This important mineral is vital for the health of our bones, teeth, muscles and heart, and our daily requirements vary with age. Help your family increase their calcium intake with these delicious meal ideas.

BREAKFAST

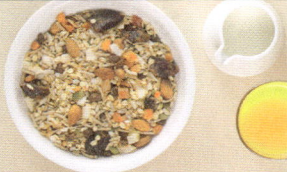 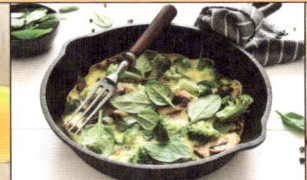 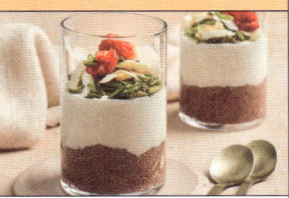

CEREAL AND JUICE Serve a bowl of calcium-fortified wholegrain cereal or muesli with milk, and a glass of orange juice on the side.

OMELETTE Whisk eggs and cook gently in a frypan on one side. Add cheese, mushrooms and spinach, fold and cook through.

CHIA SEED PUDDING Mix 2 tablespoons chia seeds with 2/3 cup almond milk and leave to set. Serve with nuts, berries or yoghurt.

LUNCH

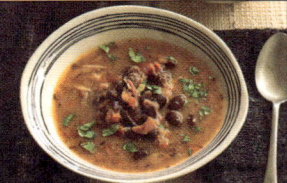 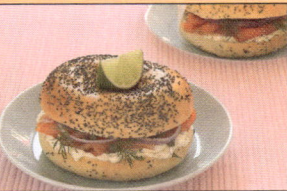 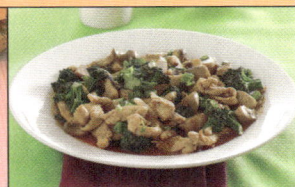

BEAN SOUP Make a hearty soup from canned beans (try lentils, white beans or black beans), vegetables and spices. Enjoy with grainy bread.

SMOKED SALMON BAGEL Spread a sesame or poppy seed bagel with cream cheese and smoked salmon for a delicious and filling option.

STIR-FRY Enjoy a tasty chicken and broccoli stir-fry with a splash of sesame oil, swapping the chicken for tofu if you're vegetarian.

DINNER

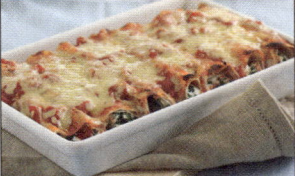 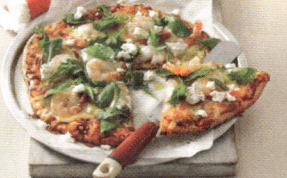 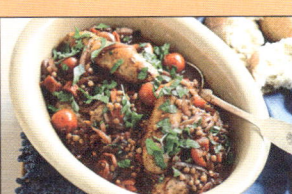

SPINACH & RICOTTA CANNELLONI Fill cannelloni tubes with a mixture of ricotta, mozzarella and spinach for a triple dose of calcium.

PRAWN PIZZA Make your own flatbread from flour and Greek yoghurt, then top with prawns, fetta and rocket for a healthy takeaway alternative.

SAUSAGE & LENTIL CASSEROLE Boost the calcium intake of sausages by pairing with lentils, tomatoes and silverbeet.

For more information, visit Healthy Bones Australia; healthybonesaustralia.org.au

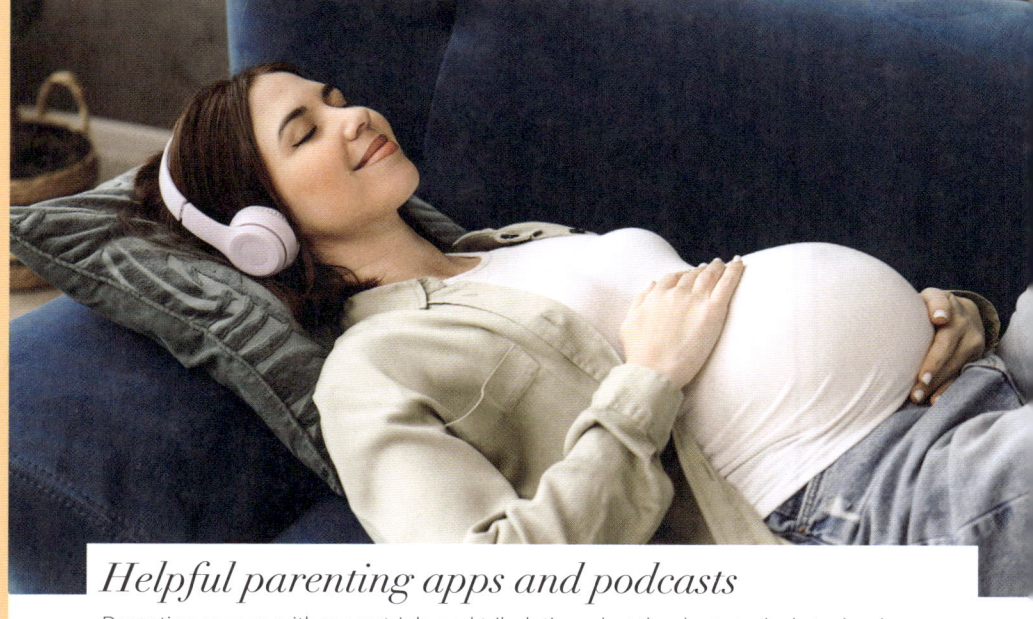

Helpful parenting apps and podcasts

Parenting comes with many trials and tribulations, but thanks to today's technology, there are some wonderful apps and podcasts to help you navigate them.

DOWNLOAD…

HEALTHDIRECT Check your symptoms, find health services near you, read up on health conditions and medications and more in this government-funded app.

SLEEP NINJA Developed by the Black Dog Institute, this adolescent-focused app teaches teens strategies to improve sleep quality and adopt healthy sleep habits.

ST JOHN FIRST RESPONDER Provides first aid support, shows all defibrillators near you and sends your location to Triple Zero (000) if you call for an ambulance.

ABA MUM2MUM Find answers to common breastfeeding questions, log your baby's sleep, feeding and changing patterns and search for breastfeeding rooms near you.

FOODSWITCH Use your phone camera to scan the barcode of a packaged food to see its Health Star Rating and find healthier 'switch' suggestions for your family.

LISTEN…

PARENTAL AS ANYTHING Parenting educator Maggie Dent and teen specialist Bec Sparrow share practical solutions to some of parenting's biggest challenges.

HAPPY FAMILIES Parenting expert and dad-of-six Dr Justin Coulson brings a common-sense approach to parenting, with daily episodes aimed at time-poor parents.

RAISING LEARNERS Presented by Raising Children Network, episodes offer practical ways to support your child's learning, from internet safety to social development.

SUE LARKEY As a teacher who specialises in special education, Sue shares strategies for supporting children with Autism Spectrum Disorder and other diagnoses at school.

THE SCIENCE OF MOTHERHOOD Doula and biochemist Dr Renee White interviews scientists and thought leaders on the latest pregnancy, birth and mothercare research.

Children and mobile phones

Whether you're contemplating getting your child a mobile phone or they already have one, there are a number of pros and pitfalls around phone use that parents will need to manage. On the plus side, phones can help children stay connected, provide access to information and teach them responsibility. On the downside, they can expose children to cyberbullying, inappropriate content and scams. Find the right balance with these tips.

HOW TO MANAGE YOUR CHILD'S MOBILE PHONE USE

- Show your child how to charge, use and store their phone safely, and how to manage their data so it doesn't run out.
- Set clear boundaries around when, where and how the phone can be used. Also make them aware of their school's rules around mobile phones and the importance of sticking to them.
- Utilise parental controls as needed to block or restrict apps, features or access to inappropriate content.
- Discuss how to be safe and respectful online, including not posting or engaging with harmful images or messages.
- Limit potentially harmful apps, such as social media apps, until your child has the emotional maturity to navigate them.
- Talk to them about the potential risk of cyber scams and teach them how to set a strong passcode, disable location services when not needed and to not answer calls or click on links from unknown numbers.
- Encourage positive phone use, such as calling a sick friend, taking photos of nature or downloading an app that supports their interests.
- Remain engaged in your child's phone use by asking them who they're speaking to, what they're watching and which games they're playing. Encourage them to come to you should anything go wrong.
- Set a good example by limiting your own phone use and enjoying regular device-free time together as a family.

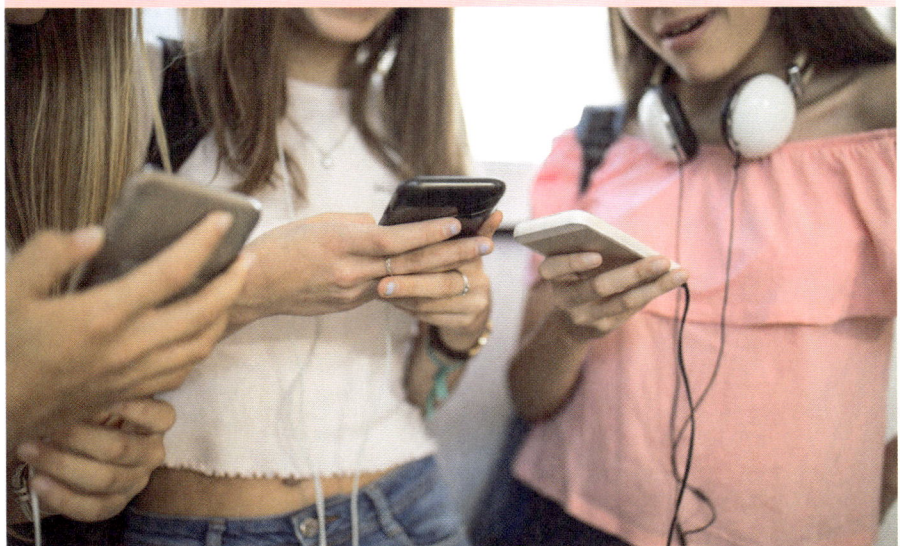

For more information, visit eSafety; esafety.gov.au

		JULY				
S	M	T	W	T	F	S
			1	2	3	4
5	6	7	8	9	10	11
12	13	14	15	16	17	18
19	20	21	22	23	24	25
26	27	28	29	30	31	

		AUGUST				
S	M	T	W	T	F	S
30	31					1
2	3	4	5	6	7	8
9	10	11	12	13	14	15
16	17	18	19	20	21	22
23	24	25	26	27	28	29

		SEPTEMBER				
S	M	T	W	T	F	S
		1	2	3	4	5
6	7	8	9	10	11	12
13	14	15	16	17	18	19
20	21	22	23	24	25	26
27	28	29	30			

3 MONDAY BANK HOLIDAY (NSW), PICNIC DAY (NT)

4 TUESDAY

5 WEDNESDAY

6 THURSDAY

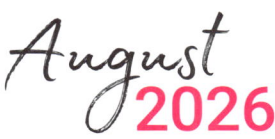

7 FRIDAY

8 SATURDAY

PRE-ORDER YOUR 2027 DIARY TODAY to unlock a special offer. Visit breastcancertrials.org.au/pre-register-diary and add a few copies for friends and family, too.

9 SUNDAY

		J	U L	Y		
S	M	T	W	T	F	S
			1	2	3	4
5	6	7	8	9	10	11
12	13	14	15	16	17	18
19	20	21	22	23	24	25
26	27	28	29	30	31	

		A U	G U	S T		
S	M	T	W	T	F	S
30	31					1
2	3	4	5	6	7	8
9	10	11	12	13	14	15
16	17	18	19	20	21	22
23	24	25	26	27	28	29

	S E	P T E	M B	E R		
S	M	T	W	T	F	S
		1	2	3	4	5
6	7	8	9	10	11	12
13	14	15	16	17	18	19
20	21	22	23	24	25	26
27	28	29	30	31		

10 MONDAY

11 TUESDAY

12 WEDNESDAY

13 THURSDAY

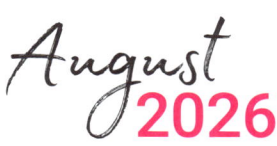

August 2026

14 FRIDAY

15 SATURDAY

PRIORITISE SELF-CARE alongside your family's needs. Enjoy regular exercise, get plenty of rest and follow your own interests.

16 SUNDAY

		J	U L Y			
S	M	T	W	T	F	S
			1	2	3	4
5	6	7	8	9	10	11
12	13	14	15	16	17	18
19	20	21	22	23	24	25
26	27	28	29	30	31	

		A U G	U S T			
S	M	T	W	T	F	S
30	31					1
2	3	4	5	6	7	8
9	10	11	12	13	14	15
16	17	18	19	20	21	22
23	24	25	26	27	28	29

		S E P T	E M B E R			
S	M	T	W	T	F	S
		1	2	3	4	5
6	7	8	9	10	11	12
13	14	15	16	17	18	19
20	21	22	23	24	25	26
27	28	29	30	31		

17 MONDAY

18 TUESDAY

19 WEDNESDAY

20 THURSDAY

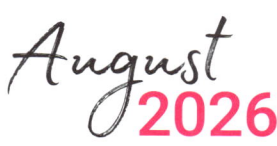

August 2026

21 FRIDAY

22 SATURDAY

INVOLVE TEENS IN FAMILY DECISIONS, especially when setting rules or boundaries around technology, bedtimes and household chores.

23 SUNDAY

	J U L Y					
S	M	T	W	T	F	S
			1	2	3	4
5	6	7	8	9	10	11
12	13	14	15	16	17	18
19	20	21	22	23	24	25
26	27	28	29	30	31	

	A U G U S T					
S	M	T	W	T	F	S
30	31					1
2	3	4	5	6	7	8
9	10	11	12	13	14	15
16	17	18	19	20	21	22
23	24	25	26	27	28	29

	S E P T E M B E R					
S	M	T	W	T	F	S
		1	2	3	4	5
6	7	8	9	10	11	12
13	14	15	16	17	18	19
20	21	22	23	24	25	26
27	28	29	30	31		

24 MONDAY

25 TUESDAY   EID MILAD UN NABI (PROPHET'S BIRTHDAY)

26 WEDNESDAY

27 THURSDAY

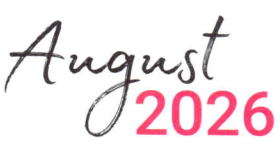

August 2026

28 FRIDAY

29 SATURDAY

> **MAKE TIME FOR YOUR PARTNER** to set a positive example for your children. Have open conversations, prioritise alone time and plan regular date nights.

30 SUNDAY

WHY I SUPPORT BREAST CANCER TRIALS

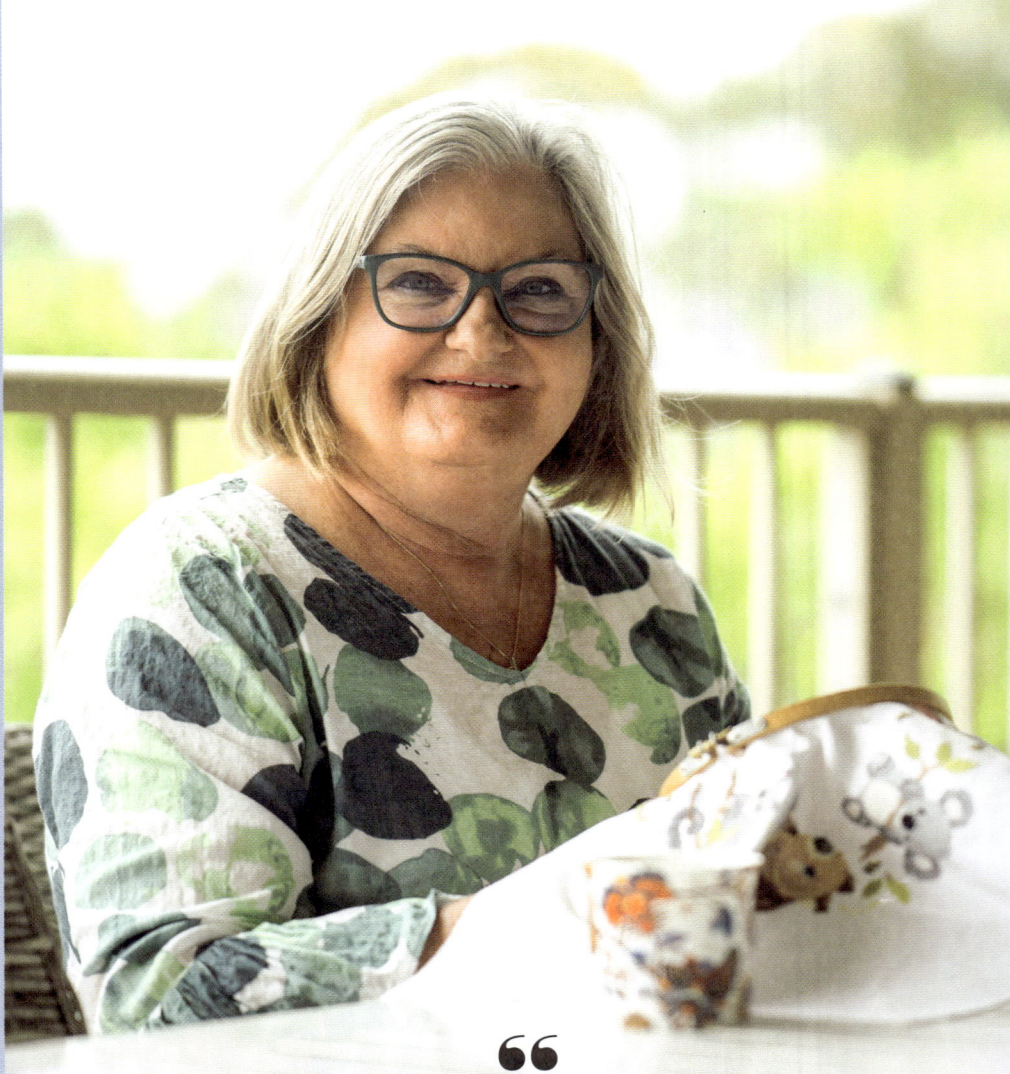

> "I had two-yearly screening mammograms and about six months after the last one I found a lump. I'm so glad I got it checked out. I hope that by being in a clinical trial I'm helping myself and other women too. You want to be here for all the moments in your family's life, and I have a grandson now. Everyone wants the future they've planned.

Wendy Rolls, diagnosed age 63

let's talk about WELLBEING

From sleep and diet to exercise and age, there are a number of factors that can boost or inhibit our mental wellbeing. Discover potential pitfalls and strategies in this chapter for a more positive experience overall.

You may be familiar with the term 'trigger': a person, place or situation linked to a past traumatic event that can bring about a negative emotional response. But did you know there are also little sensory cues – called 'glimmers' – which can spark joy, happiness, safety and connection? Glimmers are different for everyone and you may not always be aware of them. Identifying yours can have a positive impact on mental health and wellbeing, and can also give you a more compassionate and altruistic view on life.

HOW TO FIND YOUR GLIMMERS

Surrounding yourself with glimmers can assist in regulating mood, create a sense of calm and safety and help you to live without fear. But first you need to identify what your glimmers are. Start by paying attention to those moments when you feel at ease and try to pinpoint what might be happening around you to cause that feeling. Tune into your senses – what are you seeing, smelling, touching, hearing or tasting? Are you in a particular place or with a special someone?

Glimmers generally take place in the present, so practise mindfulness, meditation or breathing exercises to stay grounded and present in the moment. You might like to start a journal where you can write down your glimmers and reflect on how they make you feel.

Examples of glimmers
- Patting or cuddling a pet
- The smell of a flower, food or fragrance
- Moments in nature, such as freshly cut grass or a beautiful sunset
- The melody or lyrics of a favourite song
- Swimming in the ocean, digging in the garden or walking in the rain
- A smile or compliment from a stranger
- A memory or photograph
- Solving a crossword or ticking off a task
- Helping others.

WHAT ARE YOURS? Write down your glimmers here.

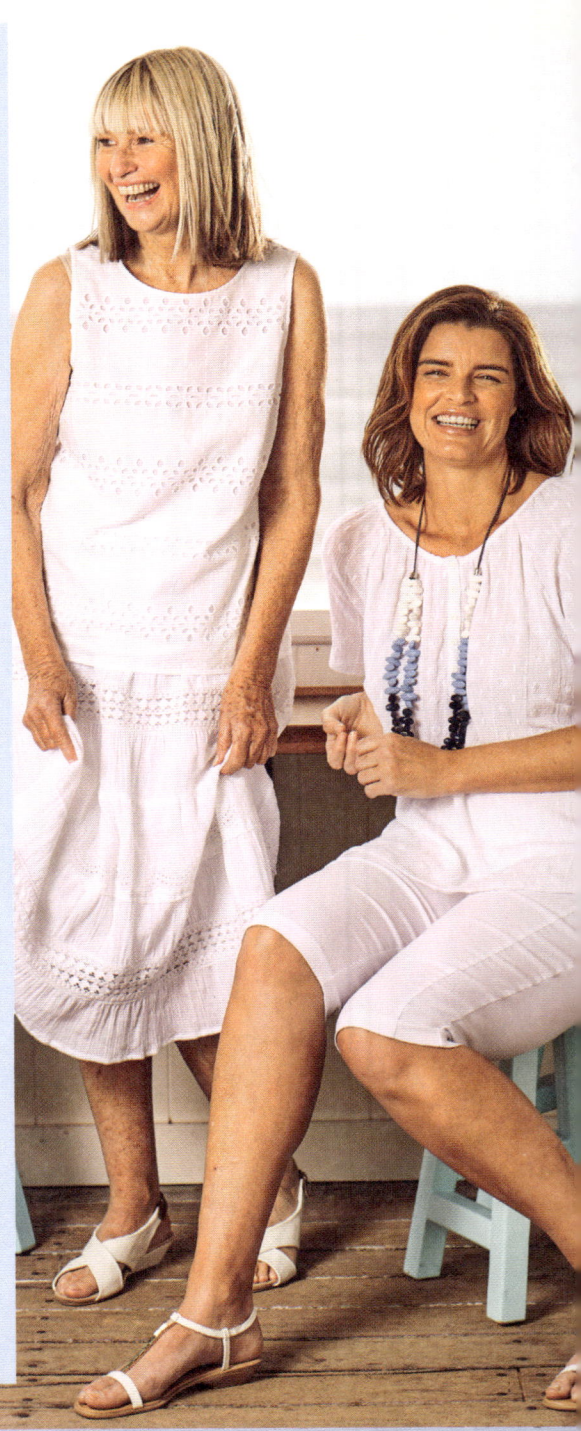

The art of friendship

Social connections are just as important for our wellbeing as exercise or a healthy diet. For some, friendships are hard to find or initiate. Try these steps – known as the 5-3-1 rule – to flex your social muscles.

5 Spend time with 5 different people each week

This can include friends, family members, colleagues, neighbours or casual acquaintances. Variety counts, so try for a mixture of interactions, from coffee dates to walk-and-talks or quick chats at the letterbox or school gate. Expand your social circle by joining clubs or groups based on your interests, signing up to volunteer or asking friends for introductions.

3 Nurture 3 close friendships

While casual interactions can help keep loneliness at bay, we also need deeper relationships with people who know us well. These are your emergency contacts or people that you often send messages to or seek out for company. Put the time and effort into maintaining these more substantial relationships by planning regular catch-ups and check-ins.

1 Enjoy 1 hour of social interaction each day

Make time every day to engage with someone in a meaningful way. Call your mum to ask about her day, join in work discussions, message a friend you haven't spoken to for a while, chat to someone on the bus or invite your neighbour for a cuppa.

Hormones and mood

Hormones are chemical substances that help control or regulate our bodily functions, behaviour, personality and emotions. We have more than 50 hormones in our body, each with their own special function. Get to know the hormones that affect our mood in different ways.

SEROTONIN Found in the brain and intestines, serotonin can affect digestion, nausea, sleep, wound healing and mood. Low levels may be associated with anxiety, depression and phobias, as well as obsessive-compulsive disorder, post-traumatic stress disorder and schizophrenia.

DOPAMINE Released by the brain, dopamine assists with gut and immune system function and is also linked with happiness, focus and motivation. Low levels may cause mood swings, memory loss and sleep problems, while high levels can lead to poor impulse control or aggression.

CORTISOL Produced by the adrenal gland, cortisol can suppress inflammation, regulate blood pressure and blood glucose levels, assist with sleep and control the body's response to stressful situations. Excess amounts of cortisol can contribute to anxiety and stress-related disorders.

PROGESTERONE Produced in the glands, ovaries and placenta, progesterone plays a role in female reproductive function, such as pregnancy, lactation and menstruation. Low levels may cause irregular periods, difficulties conceiving, troubled sleep, mood changes, pregnancy complications and contribute to menopausal symptoms.

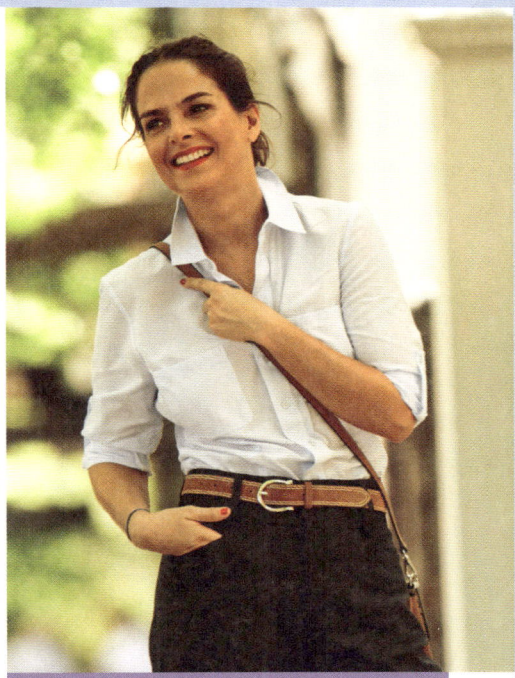

STRIKING THE RIGHT BALANCE
If you're experiencing changes in your menstrual cycle, energy levels, mood or weight, it's important to seek professional medical help. Your doctor may run tests, prescribe medication or recommend lifestyle changes, including:

Aim for 7-9 hours of quality sleep per night

Practise relaxation techniques like yoga, meditation, deep breathing or massage

Do 30 minutes of moderate-intensity exercise each day

Limit caffeine intake to one cup a day

Get 10-15 minutes of sunlight each day

Participate in hobbies that make you feel happy, relaxed and fulfilled.

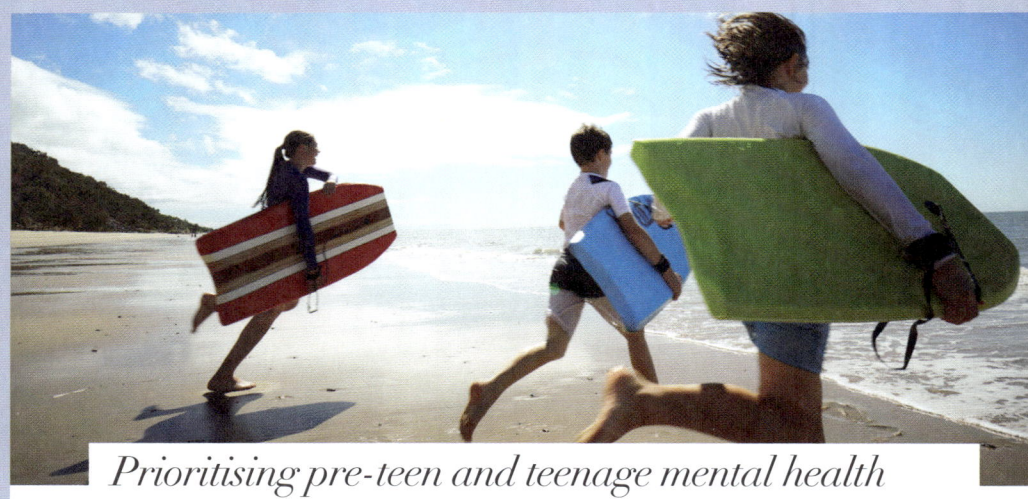

Prioritising pre-teen and teenage mental health

Adolescence can be a tricky stage for some children, throwing out a number of changes and challenges in a short amount of time. As parents and grandparents, we can help them navigate life in a positive way and look for the signs when they may be struggling.

THE WARNING SIGNS OF POOR MENTAL HEALTH

For children younger than 12 years

- Feeling sad a lot of the time
- A drop in school performance
- Ongoing worries or fears
- Loss of appetite
- Problems fitting in or getting along with other children
- Behaviour that's consistently irritable, destructive, aggressive, angry or violent
- Sleep problems, including nightmares
- Talking about self-harm or death.

For children 12 years and older

- Feeling hopeless or lacking motivation
- An inability to cope with everyday activities
- Sudden changes in behaviour for no obvious reason
- A change in appetite or sleep patterns
- Skipping school, fighting, stealing or getting in trouble
- Avoiding friends and social contact
- Weight loss or gain or anxiety around their weight or appearance
- Thoughts of self-harm or suicide.

HOW TO PROMOTE GOOD MENTAL HEALTH AND WELLBEING IN CHILDREN

- Show them love and affection in ways that they like (hugs, smiles, pats on the back).
- Take an interest in their life, praise their efforts and listen to their ideas and opinions.
- Spend one-on-one time together as well as time as a family.
- Encourage them to talk to you or another trusted adult about their problems and feelings.
- Help them to prioritise regular physical activity, healthy eating habits and a good sleep routine.
- Balance screen time and technology with other activities.
- Teach them some relaxation techniques, such as deep breathing or mindfulness.

IF YOU'RE CONCERNED ABOUT YOUR CHILD'S MENTAL HEALTH, start by talking to them about their feelings, telling them they're not alone and you're here to help. You may also need to seek professional support – see the options on the next page.

For more information, visit Headspace; headspace.org.au

Where to turn to for help

Life is full of ups and downs, but when the bad days outnumber the good, or negative thoughts persist for two weeks or more, it may help to speak to a professional. But who should you turn to? Here, we explore the range of mental health supports available to adults and children, including face-to-face, over the phone and online options.

GENERAL PRACTITIONER

Usually the first port of call, a GP can diagnose anxiety, depression and other mental health conditions, discuss treatment options, prescribe medication and refer you to a mental health professional, like a psychiatrist. They can also write you a mental health treatment plan, for access to individual or group mental health services at a reduced cost.

PSYCHOLOGIST

A registered health professional who can diagnose and treat mental health conditions, such as anxiety, depression, stress and eating disorders. Treatment or therapy – such as cognitive behavioural therapy (CBT), problem-solving therapy or interpersonal psychotherapy (IPT) – is often conducted over a period of weeks or months, with the aim of reducing the distress associated with the condition.

PSYCHIATRIST

Your GP may refer you to a psychiatrist if your anxiety or depression is severe or if you're experiencing thoughts of self-harm or suicide. Psychiatrists can also prescribe medication.

COUNSELLOR

As well as supporting people with mental health concerns, a counsellor can assist those experiencing relationship difficulties, grief or addiction. You can access counselling over the phone and online through accredited providers.

GROUPS AND FORUMS

In addition to the options mentioned, you may like to connect with others via a support group or anonymous online forum. Choose one that's facilitated by an accredited mental health organisation (such as Beyond Blue or SANE Australia) or, in the case of online forums, moderated 24/7 by mental health professionals.

CALL THESE NUMBERS FOR URGENT SUPPORT

Crisis support and suicide prevention
Lifeline Australia, 13 11 14

Youth mental health support
Kids Helpline, 1800 55 1800

Aboriginal and Torres Strait Islanders
13 YARN (13 92 76)

Alcohol and drug addiction
National Alcohol and Other Drug Hotline, 1800 250 015

Gambling
Gambling Help Line, 1800 858 858

Domestic and sexual violence
1800RESPECT (1800 737 732)

Financial support
National Debt Helpline, 1800 007 007

LGBTIQA+ individuals
QLife, 1800 184 527

If you or someone close to you is experiencing an emergency, or is at immediate risk of harm, please call Triple Zero (000).

	AUGUST					
S	M	T	W	T	F	S
30	31					1
2	3	4	5	6	7	8
9	10	11	12	13	14	15
16	17	18	19	20	21	22
23	24	25	26	27	28	29

	SEPTEMBER					
S	M	T	W	T	F	S
		1	2	3	4	5
6	7	8	9	10	11	12
13	14	15	16	17	18	19
20	21	22	23	24	25	26
27	28	29	30			

	OCTOBER					
S	M	T	W	T	F	S
				1	2	3
4	5	6	7	8	9	10
11	12	13	14	15	16	17
18	19	20	21	22	23	24
25	26	27	28	29	30	31

31 MONDAY

1 TUESDAY

2 WEDNESDAY

3 THURSDAY

September 2026

4 FRIDAY

5 SATURDAY

LISTEN TO BREAST CANCER TRIALS' PODCAST to hear the latest research findings, treatment options and stories from people impacted by breast cancer. Find it on your favourite podcast platform.

6 SUNDAY FATHER'S DAY

	AUGUST					
S	M	T	W	T	F	S
30	31					1
2	3	4	5	6	7	8
9	10	11	12	13	14	15
16	17	18	19	20	21	22
23	24	25	26	27	28	29

	SEPTEMBER					
S	M	T	W	T	F	S
		1	2	3	4	5
6	7	8	9	10	11	12
13	14	15	16	17	18	19
20	21	22	23	24	25	26
27	28	29	30			

	OCTOBER					
S	M	T	W	T	F	S
				1	2	3
4	5	6	7	8	9	10
11	12	13	14	15	16	17
18	19	20	21	22	23	24
25	26	27	28	29	30	31

7 MONDAY

8 TUESDAY

9 WEDNESDAY

10 THURSDAY R U OK? DAY

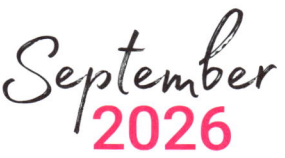
September 2026

11 FRIDAY

12 SATURDAY ROSH HASHANAH (JEWISH NEW YEAR)

BOOK A MENTAL HEALTH CHECK with your GP. Ask for a longer or double appointment, and jot down your thoughts and any questions ahead of time.

13 SUNDAY

		AUGUST				
S	M	T	W	T	F	S
30	31					1
2	3	4	5	6	7	8
9	10	11	12	13	14	15
16	17	18	19	20	21	22
23	24	25	26	27	28	29

		SEPTEMBER				
S	M	T	W	T	F	S
		1	2	3	4	5
6	7	8	9	10	11	12
13	14	15	16	17	18	19
20	21	22	23	24	25	26
27	28	29	30			

		OCTOBER				
S	M	T	W	T	F	S
				1	2	3
4	5	6	7	8	9	10
11	12	13	14	15	16	17
18	19	20	21	22	23	24
25	26	27	28	29	30	31

14 MONDAY

15 TUESDAY

16 WEDNESDAY

17 THURSDAY

September 2026

18 FRIDAY

19 SATURDAY

STOCK UP ON FOODS RICH IN TRYPTOPHAN to help boost your feel-good serotonin levels. Try salmon, eggs, spinach, tofu, nuts and seeds.

20 SUNDAY

	AUGUST					
S	M	T	W	T	F	S
30	31					1
2	3	4	5	6	7	8
9	10	11	12	13	14	15
16	17	18	19	20	21	22
23	24	25	26	27	28	29

	SEPTEMBER					
S	M	T	W	T	F	S
		1	2	3	4	5
6	7	8	9	10	11	12
13	14	15	16	17	18	19
20	21	22	23	24	25	26
27	28	29	30			

	OCTOBER					
S	M	T	W	T	F	S
				1	2	3
4	5	6	7	8	9	10
11	12	13	14	15	16	17
18	19	20	21	22	23	24
25	26	27	28	29	30	31

21 MONDAY YOM KIPPUR (JEWISH HOLY DAY)

22 TUESDAY

23 WEDNESDAY

24 THURSDAY

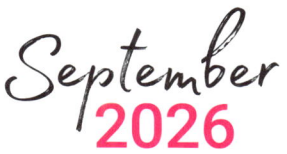
September 2026

25 FRIDAY AFL GRAND FINAL EVE (VIC)

26 SATURDAY

TREAT YOURSELF TO A MENTAL HEALTH DAY off work or household responsibilities to reduce burnout, improve mood and reduce stress.

27 SUNDAY

WHY I SUPPORT BREAST CANCER TRIALS

> My mum had breast cancer 14 years ago and I'll never forget when I told her about my diagnosis – I hope I never hear her cry like that again. We've talked about the difference in her experience to mine and how much things have changed for the better. I'm taking part in a clinical trial and hope that the future brings more advancements which will help my girls and others.
>
> Rebecca Pickering, diagnosed age 42, pictured with her family

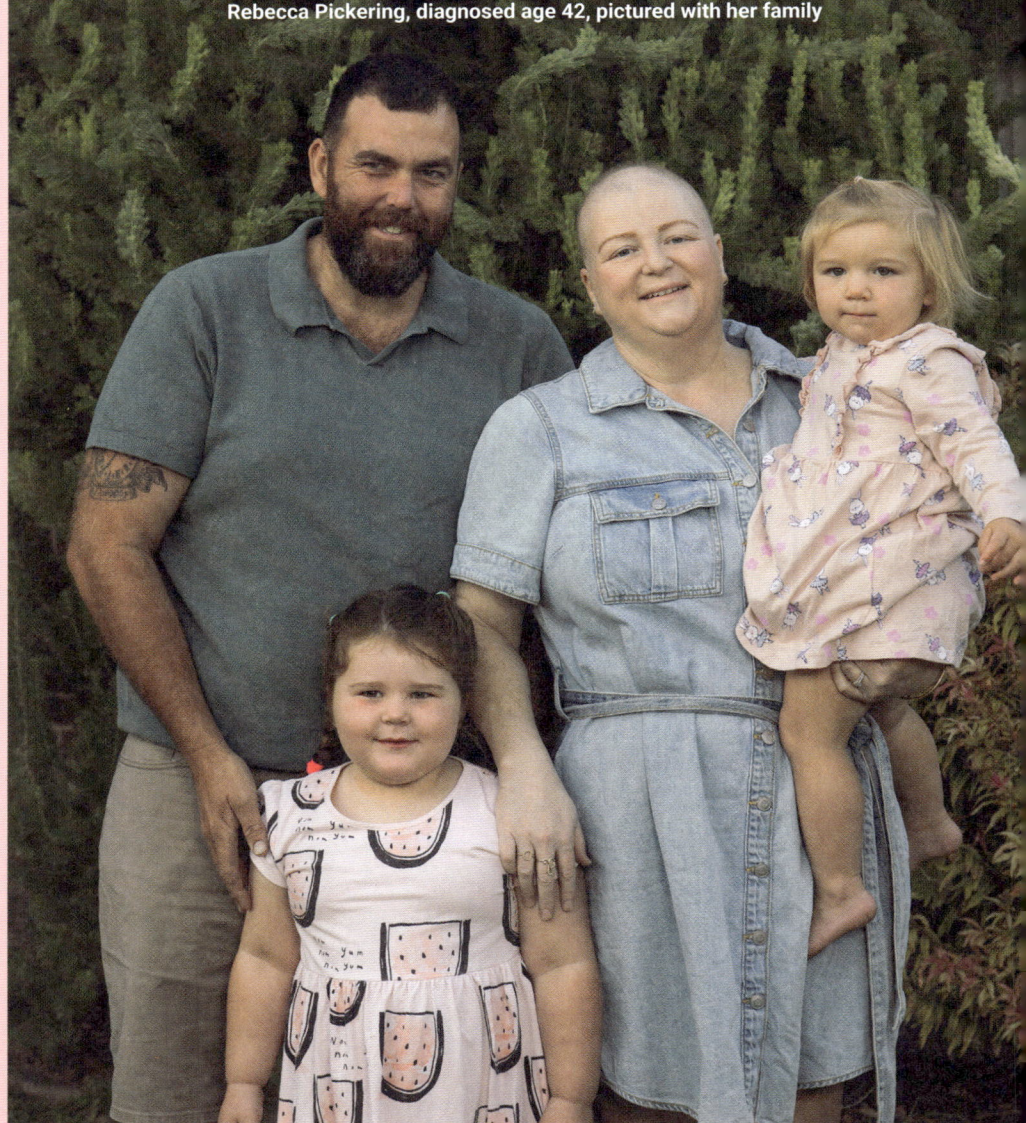

let's talk about
BREAST HEALTH

Breast cancer is so prevalent today that it's likely we all know someone who has been affected. Stay breast aware and support important research to work towards positive outcomes for every person impacted.

On average, 58 women in Australia are diagnosed with breast cancer every day and 220 men annually. Being female and increasing age are two of the main risk factors. Understand the risks and make positive changes where possible.

THE RISK FACTORS FOR BREAST CANCER

Increasing age Although breast cancer can occur in younger women, around 79 per cent of new cases are found in women over the age of 50.

Weight People who are overweight or obese have a higher risk of breast cancer than those who maintain a healthy weight. This is particularly true after menopause.

Family history Women with one or more blood relatives diagnosed with breast cancer (on their mother's or father's side) have a higher risk. As well, around 5-10 per cent of breast cancer cases are linked to an inherited gene mutation, such as BRCA1, BRCA2, PALB2 or CHEK2.

Medical history Previous exposure to chest radiation before the age of 30, long-term (more than five years) use of menopausal hormone therapy (MHT) and a previous history of breast cancer or benign breast disease can increase the risk.

Reproductive factors Periods that started before the age of 12, having children after the age of 30 or not having children and going through menopause after age 50 all pose an increased risk.

High breast density Breasts that contain a higher than average amount of fibrous and glandular tissue are associated with a higher risk.

Smoking Tobacco is a known carcinogen and smoking has been shown to increase the risk of many health conditions, including breast cancer. It can also cause complications during breast cancer treatment.

Alcohol Drinking alcohol can cause cell damage, increase hormone levels and pose a higher risk of breast cancer, with greater consumption linked with a greater risk.

HOW TO REDUCE YOUR RISK
- Eat a healthy diet
- Enjoy regular exercise
- Reduce alcohol intake
- Quit smoking
- Have regular screening mammograms
- Speak with your doctor if you have a family history of breast cancer

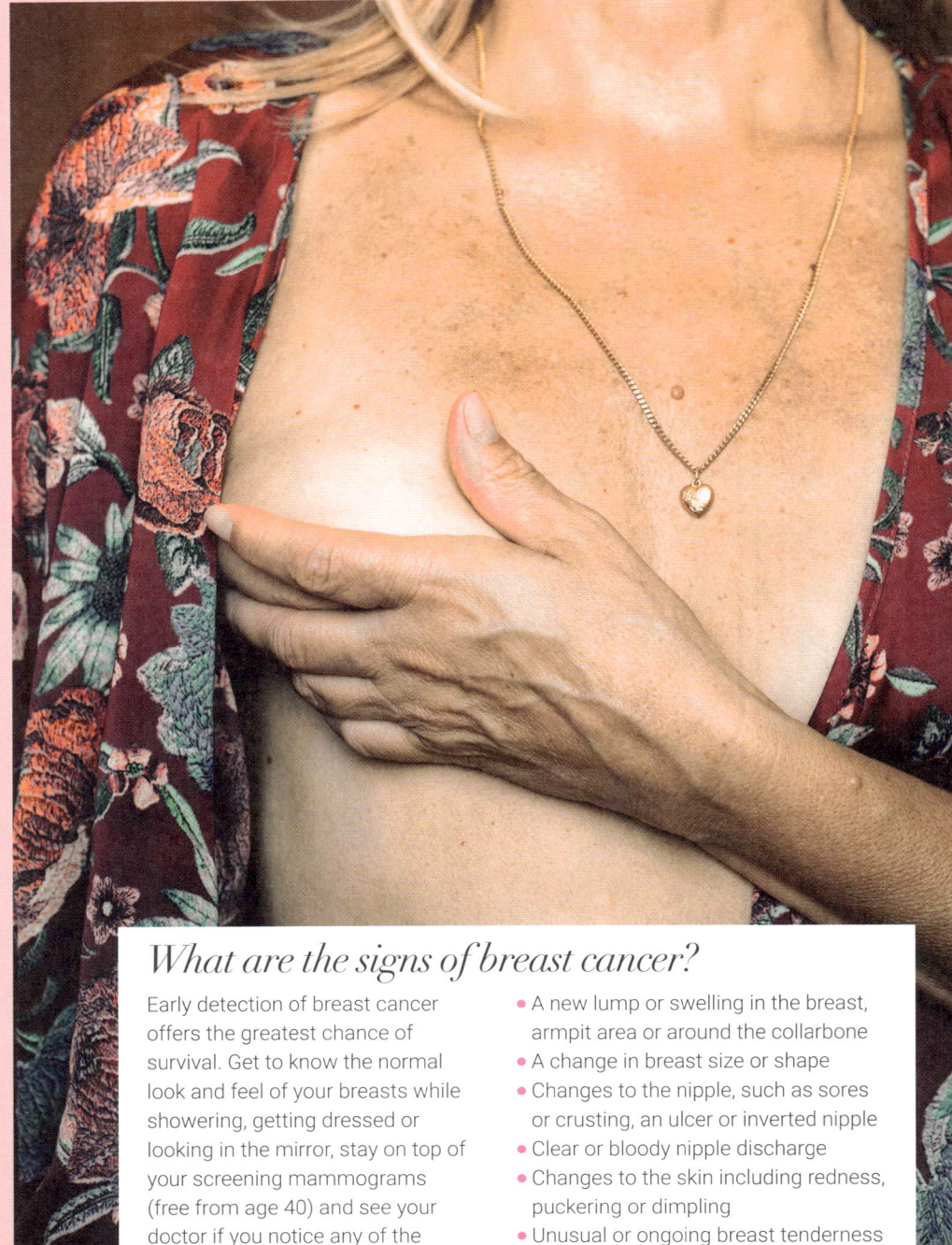

What are the signs of breast cancer?

Early detection of breast cancer offers the greatest chance of survival. Get to know the normal look and feel of your breasts while showering, getting dressed or looking in the mirror, stay on top of your screening mammograms (free from age 40) and see your doctor if you notice any of the following changes:

- A new lump or swelling in the breast, armpit area or around the collarbone
- A change in breast size or shape
- Changes to the nipple, such as sores or crusting, an ulcer or inverted nipple
- Clear or bloody nipple discharge
- Changes to the skin including redness, puckering or dimpling
- Unusual or ongoing breast tenderness or pain.

Breast cancer treatments explained

If you've received a breast cancer diagnosis, your medical team will provide guidance on the treatment options available to you. These will be tailored to individual circumstances, factoring in your age, breast cancer type, stage and location, overall health and medical history. Read on to learn more about each option and any potential side effects.

SURGERY

Treatment for early-stage breast cancer typically involves surgery to remove the breast cancer. Breast-conserving surgery (lumpectomy), involves removing the tumour and surrounding tissue while preserving the rest of the breast. Mastectomy removes the entire breast. In this case, a breast prosthesis can be used in the bra or reconstruction surgery may be offered at the same time or a later date to restore breast appearance. Mastectomy surgery can also be used as a preventative measure if you carry a gene mutation such as BRCA1, BRCA2 or PALB2, or have a strong family history of breast cancer.

CHEMOTHERAPY

This treatment is used to kill breast cancer cells that may have escaped from the breast and to prevent recurrence of early-stage breast cancer. It can also be used before surgery to shrink the size of the tumour to improve surgical outcomes, and to stop or slow the spread of cancer cells in people who have metastatic breast cancer. Drugs are administered intravenously or orally. Short-term side effects may include nausea, fatigue, hair loss, mouth ulcers, weight loss or loss of appetite. Long-term side effects can include brain 'fog', nerve damage and early menopause for younger women.

RADIOTHERAPY

Often recommended after breast-conserving surgery, radiotherapy uses localised radiation to destroy cancer cells that may remain in the breast tissue to reduce the risk of breast cancer recurrence. It may also be offered after mastectomy, depending on the stage of the cancer, and for the control of symptoms of metastatic disease. Patients may experience skin irritation, fatigue or localised swelling.

HORMONE THERAPY

For patients who have hormone receptor positive breast cancer, hormone therapy works to block or lower the level of the hormones, which are a signal for the cancer to grow. It is an effective treatment often used over several years to reduce the risk of breast cancer recurrence or control metastatic disease. Side effects can include hot flushes, mood swings, reduced libido, vaginal dryness, fatigue and joint pain.

IMMUNOTHERAPY

An emerging treatment in breast cancer, immunotherapy harnesses the body's own immune system to help fight breast cancer in its early and advanced stages. Patients who receive immunotherapy may experience a range of side effects from the immune system affecting normal tissues such as the thyroid, bowel, lungs or liver.

TARGETED THERAPY

Herceptin (trastuzumab) is a treatment for people with early-stage HER2 positive breast cancer which targets the HER2 molecule to improve survival. It is also used to stop or slow the progression of disease in people with metastatic HER2 positive breast cancer. There are other novel treatments that target specific molecules in some types of breast cancer.

How to eat and move well with breast cancer

Studies show that regular exercise and a healthy diet can reduce the risk of breast cancer. They also provide benefits if you're diagnosed with breast cancer, particularly during and after receiving treatment. Both can do wonders for your mood and energy levels, not to mention giving your body the strength and nourishment it needs to recover. But the side effects of treatment – including poor appetite, nausea and fatigue – can make this difficult. Foods may not taste the same and you might not have the energy or motivation to exercise. With advice and support from your medical team, try these ideas to do what you can.

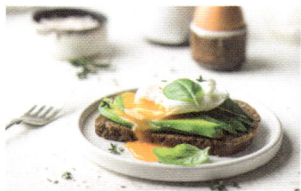

Eat when you're hungry. If you're hungrier at breakfast, make this your main meal for the day and supplement with lighter meals at other times.

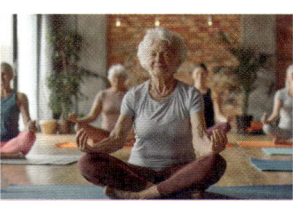

Choose gentle forms of exercise, such as Tai Chi, walking or yoga, in the weeks after treatment.

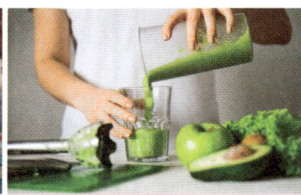

Enjoy small, frequent and nourishing drinks and snacks if your appetite is small, such as smoothies, nuts and dried fruit.

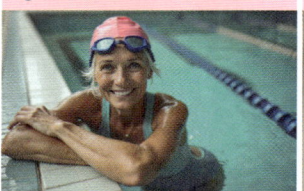

Find physical activities that you enjoy so it feels easier to accomplish your exercise goals. It might be swimming, golf or cycling.

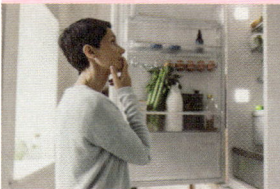

Stock your fridge and pantry with favourite foods that require minimal preparation, like peanut butter, canned tuna, cheese and eggs.

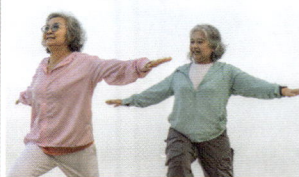

Find an exercise partner, like a friend, neighbour or family member, to keep you company.

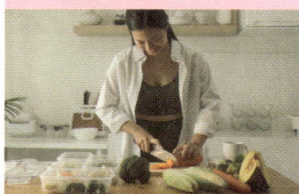

Prepare and freeze meals for the days when you don't feel like cooking. Friends and family members can help with this.

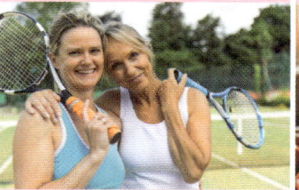

Join a class or exercise group to help you stay motivated. Try dance, Pilates or tennis.

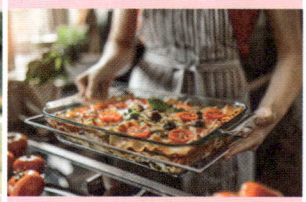

If food has a metallic taste, eat with plastic cutlery and cook in glass dishes.

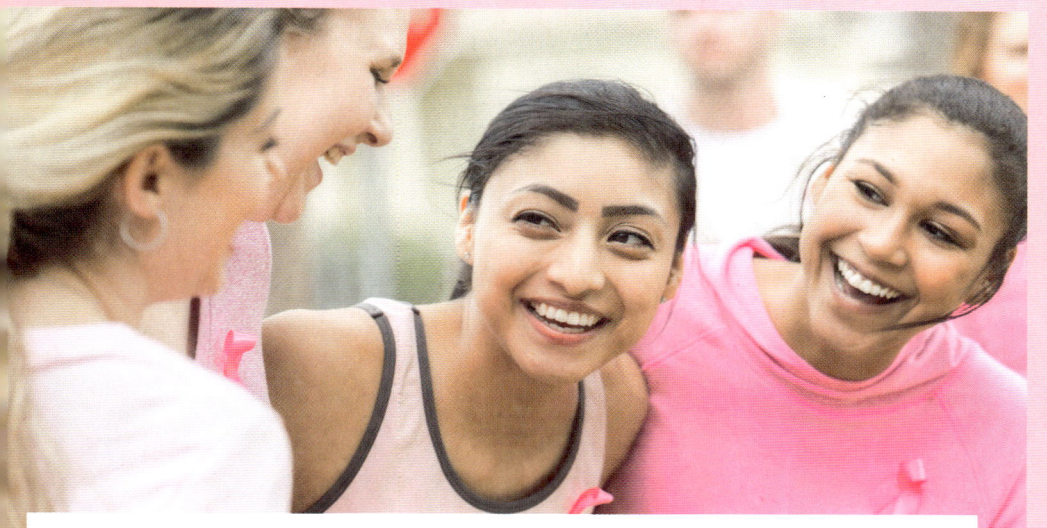

Your support saves lives

This health diary does more than help keep you organised and informed – it's also an important fundraising tool that supports the vital clinical trials research conducted by Breast Cancer Trials. Over the past 28 years, the funds raised by this diary have helped to achieve many significant advancements in the treatment and prevention of breast cancer, which are today saving the lives of women and men diagnosed. Your continued support helps to get closer to our vision of 'no more lives cut short by breast cancer'.

WHAT ARE CLINICAL TRIALS?

The clinical trials conducted by Breast Cancer Trials are carefully designed research studies aimed at identifying new and effective treatment options for every type and stage of breast cancer. Our clinical trials also aim to lessen the physical, emotional and financial burden of breast cancer on patients.

HOW DO TRIALS MAKE A DIFFERENCE?

All the breast cancer treatments currently available in Australia were first tested in clinical trials to ensure their effectiveness and safety for patients. We aim to personalise treatment to each patient's unique situation and clinical trials are the only way to achieve that. Targeting treatment and reducing side effects will result in higher survival rates and better quality of life during and after treatment.

NEW RESEARCH

Breast Cancer Trials has developed a new clinical trial called OLIO for young women diagnosed with hormone receptor positive, HER2 negative breast cancer. These patients have a poor prognosis because their breast cancer often recurs. Our researchers discovered the presence of a feature in the tumours of younger women that could be targeted with a treatment to kill the cancer cell. The trial will also test the addition of immunotherapy to help the body fight the cancer. It's hoped this treatment combination will save more lives.

For more information, visit Breast Cancer Trials; breastcancertrials.org.au

		S	E	P	T	E	M	B	E	R		

S	M	T	W	T	F	S
		1	2	3	4	5
6	7	8	9	10	11	12
13	14	15	16	17	18	19
20	21	22	23	24	25	26
27	28	29	30			

OCTOBER

S	M	T	W	T	F	S
				1	2	3
4	5	6	7	8	9	10
11	12	13	14	15	16	17
18	19	20	21	22	23	24
25	26	27	28	29	30	31

NOVEMBER

S	M	T	W	T	F	S
1	2	3	4	5	6	7
8	9	10	11	12	13	14
15	16	17	18	19	20	21
22	23	24	25	26	27	28
29	30					

28 MONDAY KING'S BIRTHDAY (WA)

29 TUESDAY

30 WEDNESDAY

1 THURSDAY BREAST CANCER AWARENESS MONTH

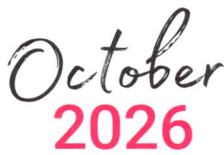
October 2026

2 FRIDAY

3 SATURDAY

HELP SAVE LIVES by purchasing your 2027 diary or making a donation to breast cancer trials research today. Visit breastcancertrials.org.au or call 1800 423 444.

4 SUNDAY   DAYLIGHT SAVING TIME BEGINS (ACT, NSW, SA, TAS, VIC)

	SEPTEMBER					
S	M	T	W	T	F	S
		1	2	3	4	5
6	7	8	9	10	11	12
13	14	15	16	17	18	19
20	21	22	23	24	25	26
27	28	29	30			

	OCTOBER					
S	M	T	W	T	F	S
					1	2
3	4	5	6	7	8	9
10	11	12	13	14	15	16
17	18	19	20	21	22	23
24	25	26	27	28	29	30
31						

	NOVEMBER					
S	M	T	W	T	F	S
	1	2	3	4	5	6
7	8	9	10	11	12	13
14	15	16	17	18	19	20
21	22	23	24	25	26	27
28	29	30				

5 MONDAY — LABOUR DAY (ACT, NSW, SA), KING'S BIRTHDAY (QLD)

6 TUESDAY

7 WEDNESDAY

8 THURSDAY

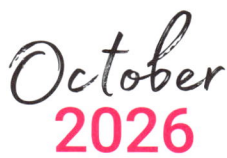
October 2026

9 FRIDAY

10 SATURDAY

SEEK ADVICE FROM YOUR GP if you're worried about your weight. They can refer you to a dietitian or help create an exercise plan to suit your age and fitness level.

11 SUNDAY

SEPTEMBER						
S	M	T	W	T	F	S
		1	2	3	4	5
6	7	8	9	10	11	12
13	14	15	16	17	18	19
20	21	22	23	24	25	26
27	28	29	30			

OCTOBER						
S	M	T	W	T	F	S
					1	2	3
4	5	6	7	8	9	10
11	12	13	14	15	16	17
18	19	20	21	22	23	24
25	26	27	28	29	30	31

NOVEMBER						
S	M	T	W	T	F	S
1	2	3	4	5	6	7
8	9	10	11	12	13	14
15	16	17	18	19	20	21
22	23	24	25	26	27	28
29	30					

12 MONDAY

13 TUESDAY

14 WEDNESDAY

15 THURSDAY

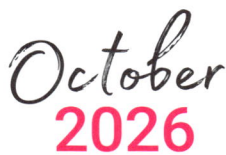
October 2026

16 FRIDAY

17 SATURDAY

> **THERE IS NO SAFE LEVEL OF ALCOHOL** when it comes to cancer risk. Have regular alcohol-free days during the week and try non-alcoholic options when socialising.

18 SUNDAY

		SEPTEMBER				
S	M	T	W	T	F	S
		1	2	3	4	5
6	7	8	9	10	11	12
13	14	15	16	17	18	19
20	21	22	23	24	25	26
27	28	29	30			

		OCTOBER				
S	M	T	W	T	F	S
				1	2	3
4	5	6	7	8	9	10
11	12	13	14	15	16	17
18	19	20	21	22	23	24
25	26	27	28	29	30	31

		NOVEMBER				
S	M	T	W	T	F	S
1	2	3	4	5	6	7
8	9	10	11	12	13	14
15	16	17	18	19	20	21
22	23	24	25	26	27	28
29	30					

19 MONDAY

20 TUESDAY

21 WEDNESDAY

22 THURSDAY ROYAL HOBART SHOW (TAS)

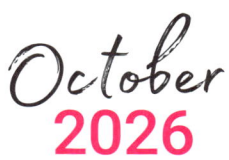
October 2026

23 FRIDAY

24 SATURDAY

IF YOU HAVE A FAMILY HISTORY of breast cancer, use the iPrevent tool to better understand what it means for you. Visit iPrevent.net.au.

25 SUNDAY

	SEPTEMBER					
S	M	T	W	T	F	S
		1	2	3	4	5
6	7	8	9	10	11	12
13	14	15	16	17	18	19
20	21	22	23	24	25	26
27	28	29	30			

	OCTOBER					
S	M	T	W	T	F	S
				1	2	3
4	5	6	7	8	9	10
11	12	13	14	15	16	17
18	19	20	21	22	23	24
25	26	27	28	29	30	31

	NOVEMBER					
S	M	T	W	T	F	S
1	2	3	4	5	6	7
8	9	10	11	12	13	14
15	16	17	18	19	20	21
22	23	24	25	26	27	28
29	30					

26 MONDAY AUSTRALIA'S BREAST CANCER DAY

27 TUESDAY

28 WEDNESDAY

29 THURSDAY

October–November 2026

30 FRIDAY

31 SATURDAY HALLOWEEN

> **STAY ON TOP OF YOUR MAMMOGRAMS.** All women aged 40 and over are eligible for a free screening mammogram every two years – call 13 20 50 to book yours today.

1 SUNDAY

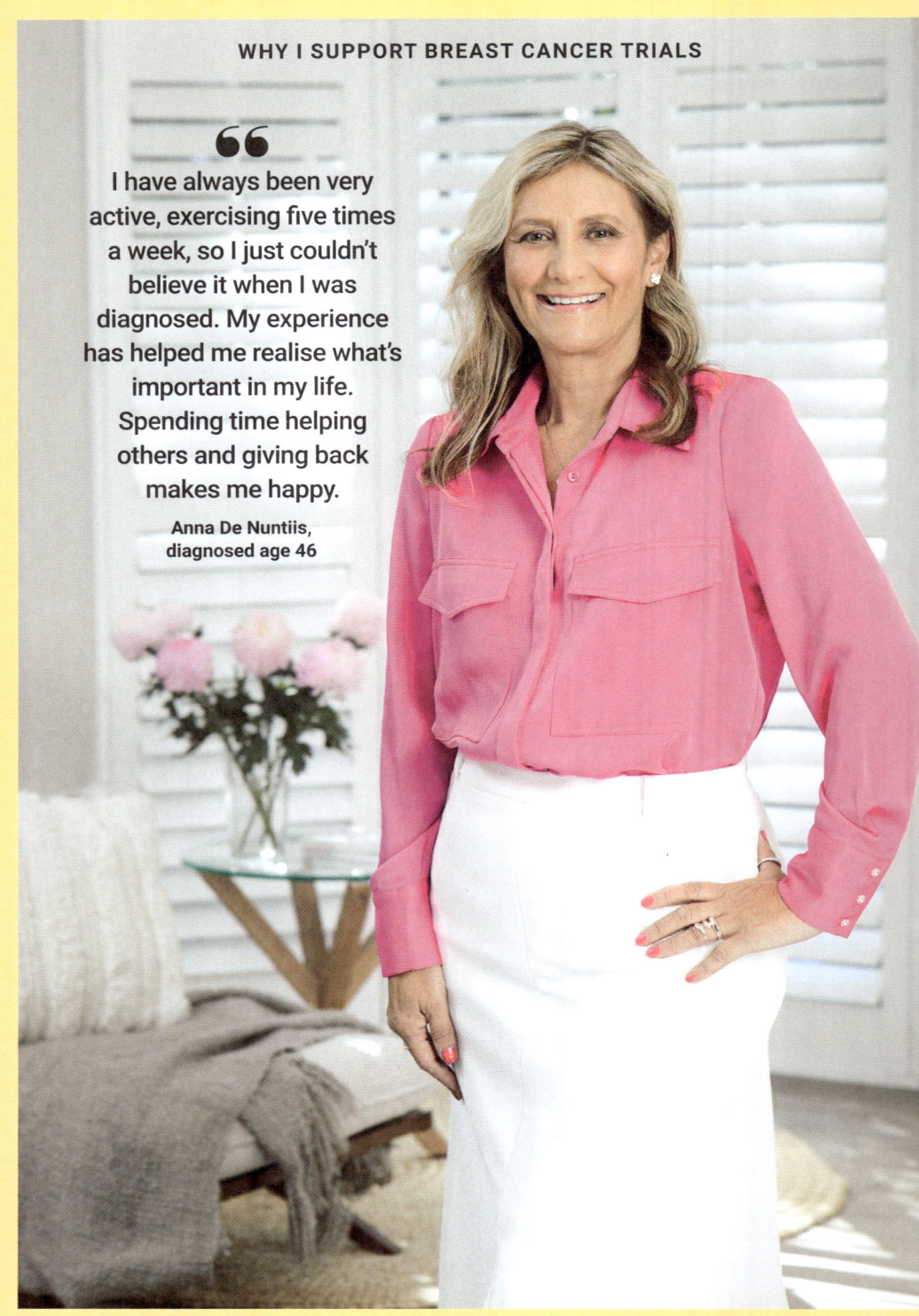

WHY I SUPPORT BREAST CANCER TRIALS

> I have always been very active, exercising five times a week, so I just couldn't believe it when I was diagnosed. My experience has helped me realise what's important in my life. Spending time helping others and giving back makes me happy.

Anna De Nuntiis, diagnosed age 46

let's talk about HEALTHY SKIN

From sun safety measures and regular spot checks to smarter lifestyle choices, learn how to take care of your skin so it can continue taking care of you.

The skin is one of our hardest-working organs, helping to regulate body temperature and protecting us from viruses and bacteria. But there are certain unhelpful habits that can have a negative impact on our skin. Put an end to these five habits for healthier skin today.

5 BAD HABITS THAT CAN HARM YOUR SKIN

1 Not drinking enough water
Skin dryness often starts below the surface when the body is dehydrated. Combat this by drinking eight cups of fluids per day. Liquids like tea, coffee, milk, juice and soup count towards your intake, but plain water is best for hydration. Help your cause by keeping bottles of water nearby – beside your bed, in the fridge, at your desk or in the car.

2 Smoking and drinking alcohol
Smoking and vaping restricts blood flow, which can accelerate the signs of ageing and lead to a dull complexion, while alcohol dehydrates the skin and may cause bloating, puffiness, acne and wrinkles. Quit smoking by visiting quit.org.au, and refer to our Lifestyle chapter for ways to reduce your alcohol consumption.

3 Eating the wrong foods
Diet plays a key role in skin health, with highly processed foods, refined carbohydrates and foods high in sugar and salt increasing the risk of acne. Include a variety of fresh fruit, vegetables and healthy fats in your diet to nourish the skin.

4 Inadequate sleep
If you're lacking in sleep, you may be more susceptible to acne breakouts, swelling, rashes and skin conditions like eczema and rosacea. In addition, your immune system can be weakened, impacting the body's ability to produce collagen and elastin for skin firmness and elasticity. To improve your sleep, try to stick to the same sleep and wake-up times each day, limit caffeine, rigorous exercise and screen time in the hours before bed and avoid naps during the day.

5 Skipping sunscreen
Forgetting to apply sunscreen to areas of the skin that are exposed to sunlight can increase our risk of developing skin cancer and lead to premature skin ageing. Make a habit of applying a broad-spectrum SPF 50+ sunscreen as part of your morning routine, regardless of the weather. Carry a tube with you for reapplication on the go.

For more information, visit The Australasian College of Dermatologists; dermcoll.edu.au

Know your skin cancer risk

Australia has one of the highest rates of skin cancer in the world. Two in three people will be diagnosed by age 70, and around 2000 will die from it each year. Our best line of defence is getting to know the normal look of our skin so we can detect any changes straightaway.

Develop a regular habit of checking your skin for new spots or changes to existing moles and freckles.

The signs of skin cancer
- A spot that looks and feels different to other spots on your skin
- A spot that has changed in size, shape, thickness, colour or texture
- A spot that is tender or sore to touch
- A sore that doesn't heal within a few weeks
- A sore that is itchy or bleeding.

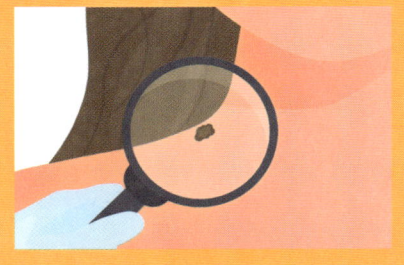

BASAL CELL CARCINOMA (BCC)
- A slow-growing, non-melanoma skin cancer, which makes up about 70 per cent of skin cancer cases.
- Very rarely spreads to other parts of the body, but if undetected, may grow deeper or invade nerves and tissue to make treatment more difficult.
- BCC can occur anywhere but is often found on sun-exposed areas like the head, neck, ears, shoulders, arms and legs.
- Look for pearly or shiny flat or raised lumps, which may become itchy or inflamed and form scabs or sores.

SQUAMOUS CELL CARCINOMA (SCC)
- The second most common non-melanoma skin cancer, which can grow quickly over a period of weeks or months and may spread to other parts of the body if untreated.
- Accounts for about one in three skin cancer cases.
- Found in the same areas as BCC.
- Look for a thick or nodular, scaly lesion, red or pink in colour, which may be itchy, bleeding, inflamed or tender to the touch.

MELANOMA
- The most serious type of skin cancer as it can grow quickly and spread to other parts of the body.
- About one in 100 skin cancers are melanoma, and there are five main melanoma subtypes.
- Can appear in areas that have been exposed to the sun and also areas that don't receive much sun, such as the eyes, nasal passages, mouth, genitals, soles of the feet, palms of the hands and under the nails.
- Look for a new or existing flat spot or mole with an uneven border, which changes in size, colour or shape (superficial spreading melanoma) or a round, raised pink, red, brown or black lump that feels firm to the touch and may bleed or have a crusty surface (nodular melanoma).

If you notice a spot that worries you, see your doctor for further investigation.

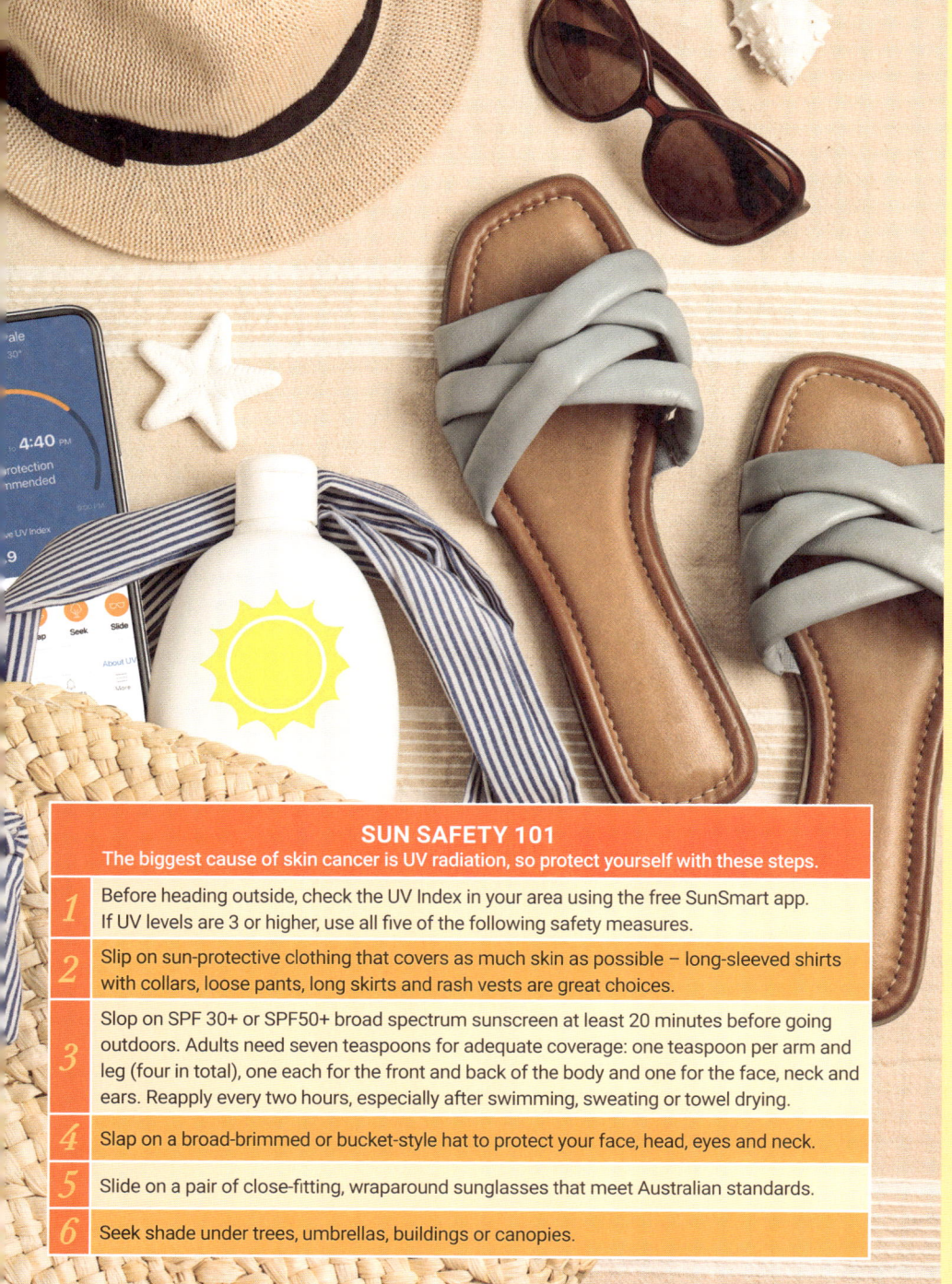

SUN SAFETY 101
The biggest cause of skin cancer is UV radiation, so protect yourself with these steps.

1	Before heading outside, check the UV Index in your area using the free SunSmart app. If UV levels are 3 or higher, use all five of the following safety measures.
2	Slip on sun-protective clothing that covers as much skin as possible – long-sleeved shirts with collars, loose pants, long skirts and rash vests are great choices.
3	Slop on SPF 30+ or SPF50+ broad spectrum sunscreen at least 20 minutes before going outdoors. Adults need seven teaspoons for adequate coverage: one teaspoon per arm and leg (four in total), one each for the front and back of the body and one for the face, neck and ears. Reapply every two hours, especially after swimming, sweating or towel drying.
4	Slap on a broad-brimmed or bucket-style hat to protect your face, head, eyes and neck.
5	Slide on a pair of close-fitting, wraparound sunglasses that meet Australian standards.
6	Seek shade under trees, umbrellas, buildings or canopies.

Your seasonal skincare guide

Ensure your skin looks radiant and healthy throughout the year with these seasonal tips.

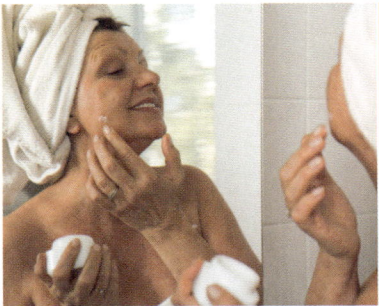

SUMMER

- Wash your face with a mild foaming or gel cleanser twice a day to remove sweat, sunscreen and excess oil.
- Even on humid days, our skin needs moisture, so opt for a lightweight moisturiser that will hydrate without feeling greasy.
- After a day spent outdoors (don't forget the Sun Safety steps), replenish the skin with after-sun products containing aloe vera and antioxidants.

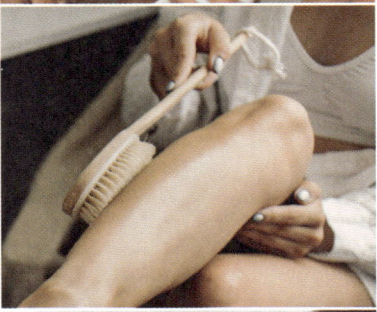

AUTUMN

- As the air becomes drier, transition to a rich, hydrating moisturiser containing ceramides or hyaluronic acid to lock in moisture.
- Our skin-shedding process tends to slow down in the colder months, so exfoliate regularly to remove dead skin and reduce clogged pores.
- Continue using sunscreen. The sun's rays may not feel as intense, but UV rays can still do damage.

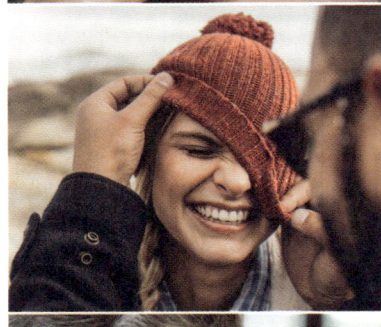

WINTER

- Avoid too-hot showers or baths, which can strip skin of essential oils and dry it out. Opt for lukewarm water instead, and limit showers to 5-10 minutes.
- Wear gloves when going outside to protect your hands from the cold, and apply a rich hand cream after washing your hands.
- Lips can be prone to cracking in winter. Protect them by regularly applying a vitamin-enriched lip balm formulated with SPF50+.

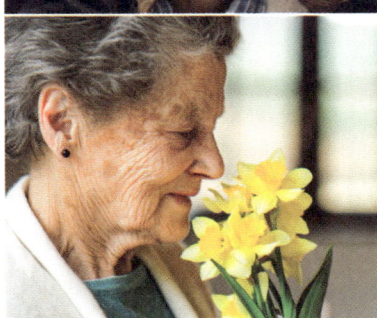

SPRING

- Seasonal allergies can trigger skin sensitivities. Look for a barrier cream containing zinc or natural oils to act as a shield against potential irritants.
- Treat redness, itching and irritation with gentle lotions or balms free of fragrances, harsh preservatives and alcohol. Cool compresses may also help.
- Give make-up brushes, loofahs and sponges a spring clean using warm water and liquid soap, then leave to dry. Dispose of any expired creams and gels.

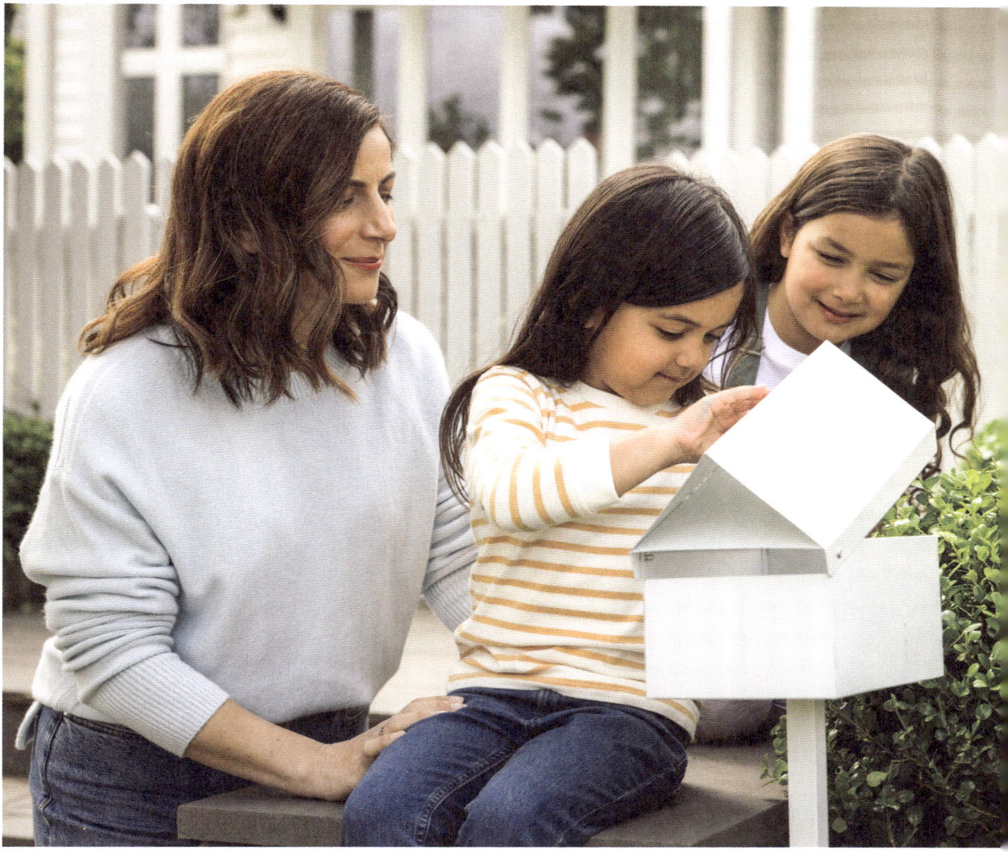

Delivering the Goods

By sending books to First Nations children, supporting mental wellbeing and raising funds in times of disaster, we're supporting communities in every corner of the country.

auspost.com.au/supportingcommunities

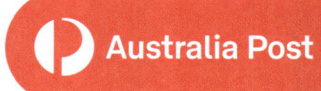 Australia Post

	OCTOBER					
S	M	T	W	T	F	S
				1	2	3
4	5	6	7	8	9	10
11	12	13	14	15	16	17
18	19	20	21	22	23	24
25	26	27	28	29	30	31

	NOVEMBER					
S	M	T	W	T	F	S
1	2	3	4	5	6	7
8	9	10	11	12	13	14
15	16	17	18	19	20	21
22	23	24	25	26	27	28
29	30					

	DECEMBER					
S	M	T	W	T	F	S
		1	2	3	4	5
6	7	8	9	10	11	12
13	14	15	16	17	18	19
20	21	22	23	24	25	26
27	28	29	30	31		

2 MONDAY RECREATION DAY (TAS)

3 TUESDAY MELBOURNE CUP DAY (VIC)

4 WEDNESDAY

5 THURSDAY

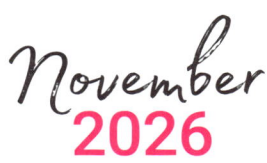
November 2026

6 FRIDAY

7 SATURDAY

ADD SOME POLYPHENOLS TO YOUR DIET to improve skin firmness and radiance and fight the signs of ageing. Get them from apples, eggplant, legumes or tea.

8 SUNDAY   DIWALI (HINDU, BUDDHIST, JAIN AND SIKH FESTIVAL)

	OCTOBER					
S	M	T	W	T	F	S
				1	2	3
4	5	6	7	8	9	10
11	12	13	14	15	16	17
18	19	20	21	22	23	24
25	26	27	28	29	30	31

	NOVEMBER					
S	M	T	W	T	F	S
1	2	3	4	5	6	7
8	9	10	11	12	13	14
15	16	17	18	19	20	21
22	23	24	25	26	27	28
29	30					

	DECEMBER					
S	M	T	W	T	F	S
		1	2	3	4	5
6	7	8	9	10	11	12
13	14	15	16	17	18	19
20	21	22	23	24	25	26
27	28	29	30	31		

9 MONDAY

10 TUESDAY

11 WEDNESDAY REMEMBRANCE DAY

12 THURSDAY

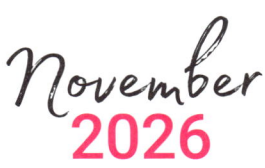
November 2026

13 FRIDAY

14 SATURDAY

> **CHANGE YOUR PILLOWCASE** once a week. The oil from your hair can leave a residue that transfers to your skin while you sleep.

15 SUNDAY

		OCTOBER				
S	M	T	W	T	F	S
				1	2	3
4	5	6	7	8	9	10
11	12	13	14	15	16	17
18	19	20	21	22	23	24
25	26	27	28	29	30	31

		NOVEMBER				
S	M	T	W	T	F	S
1	2	3	4	5	6	7
8	9	10	11	12	13	14
15	16	17	18	19	20	21
22	23	24	25	26	27	28
29	30					

		DECEMBER				
S	M	T	W	T	F	S
		1	2	3	4	5
6	7	8	9	10	11	12
13	14	15	16	17	18	19
20	21	22	23	24	25	26
27	28	29	30	31		

16 MONDAY

17 TUESDAY

18 WEDNESDAY

19 THURSDAY

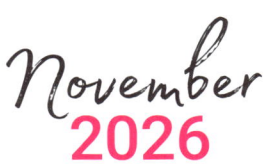
November 2026

20 FRIDAY

21 SATURDAY

LEAVE A GIFT IN YOUR WILL to help create a future where breast cancer no longer impacts lives. For more information visit breastcancertrials.org.au or call 1800 423 444.

22 SUNDAY

	OCTOBER					
S	M	T	W	T	F	S
				1	2	3
4	5	6	7	8	9	10
11	12	13	14	15	16	17
18	19	20	21	22	23	24
25	26	27	28	29	30	31

	NOVEMBER					
S	M	T	W	T	F	S
1	2	3	4	5	6	7
8	9	10	11	12	13	14
15	16	17	18	19	20	21
22	23	24	25	26	27	28
29	30					

	DECEMBER					
S	M	T	W	T	F	S
		1	2	3	4	5
6	7	8	9	10	11	12
13	14	15	16	17	18	19
20	21	22	23	24	25	26
27	28	29	30	31		

23 MONDAY

24 TUESDAY

25 WEDNESDAY

26 THURSDAY

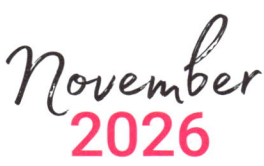
November 2026

27 FRIDAY

28 SATURDAY

> **PROTECT YOUR BABY'S SKIN** by staying indoors when the UV Index is 3 or above. When outdoors, cover their skin with loose-fitting clothing, a hat and a pram shade cover.

29 SUNDAY

WHY I SUPPORT BREAST CANCER TRIALS

I never realised there were different types of breast cancer until I was diagnosed. I have participated in two clinical trials, one of which is testing if a new medication is more effective at preventing breast cancer recurring than current treatments. I hope my participation will help future people diagnosed.

Elissa Simms, diagnosed age 48

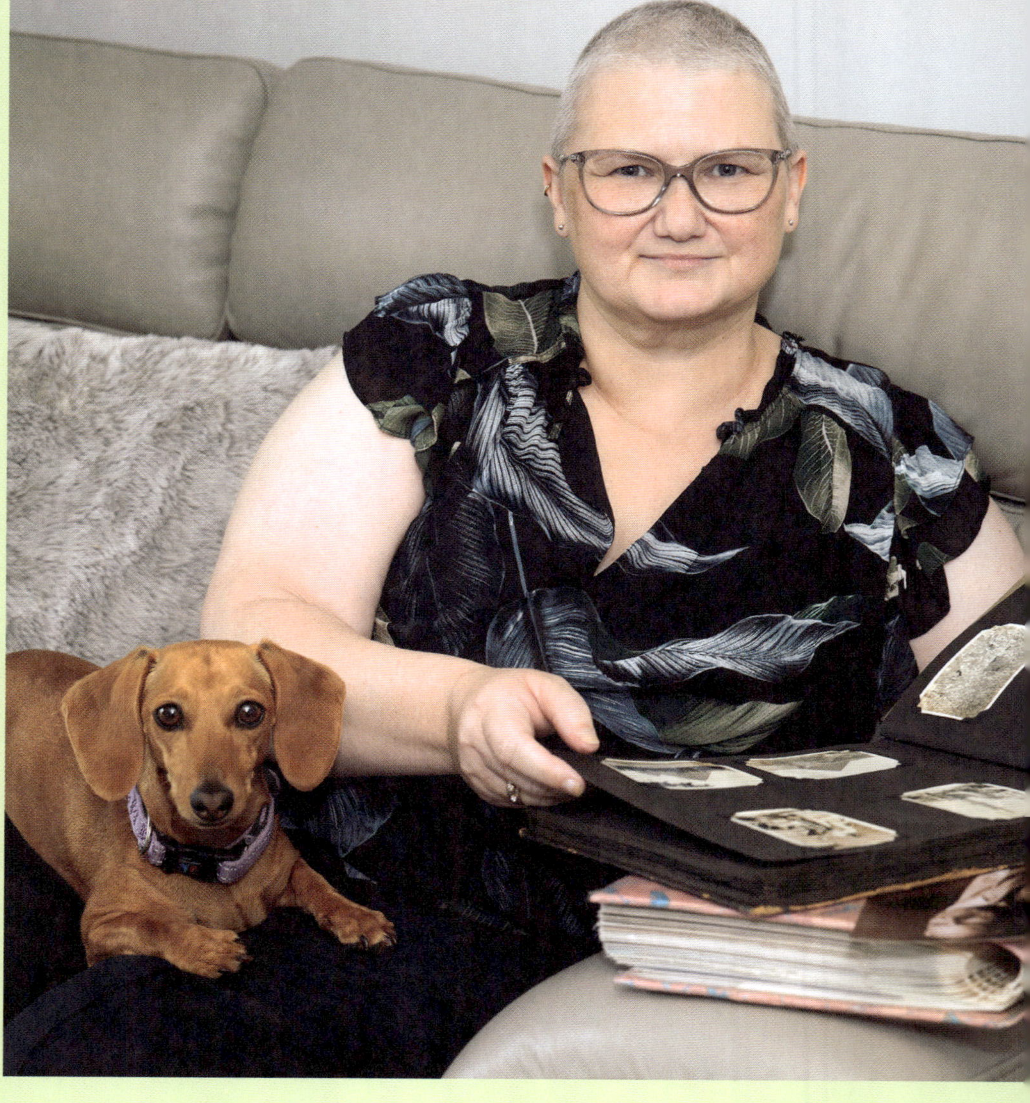

let's talk about LIFESTYLE

Finish the year by taking a holistic approach to your health. Consider all aspects of your lifestyle to achieve happiness, vitality and start the next year stronger than ever.

As the end of the year approaches, many Australians will take a well-earned break over summer. During this period, our healthy habits can often lapse. While the odd sleep-in or cheat day won't do any lasting damage, long periods of holiday excess can have a negative impact on our health and wellbeing. Enjoy your downtime while continuing with your health goals using these tips.

STAY ACTIVE

It can be difficult sticking with your normal exercise routine when days lack their usual structure. Embrace the change in routine and find new ways to get moving. Check out the hotel gym, plan a day of sightseeing on foot, swim laps at the local pool or exercise with friends.

EAT WELL

Socialising over the silly season often coincides with a meal, while holidays offer opportunities to eat out more or sample the delights at the breakfast buffet. The trick is to allow yourself these treats while making healthy choices to balance it out. Watch your portion sizes and opt for salads, antipasti, grilled lean meats and fresh seafood over deep-fried, salt-laden or sugary options.

MANAGE SLEEP

Between entertaining, socialising and travelling, it can be hard to maintain our regular sleep patterns. Try planning social catch-ups around the middle of the day so as not to interfere with your usual sleep and wake times, avoid the temptation to sleep late or nap for long periods and reduce the effects of jet lag by adjusting your sleep-wake times by 20 to 30 minutes every few days in the weeks before your trip.

A flexible routine is key to enjoying some well-earned respite without derailing all of your health intentions.

SWITCH OFF

Time away from work, school or your usual routine may leave you with extra hours to fill, and it can be tempting to get comfortable binge-watching your favourite show or give the kids more screen time. Limit sedentary time to an hour here or there and plan some screen-free activities in between, such as cooking, bike rides, bush walks or trips to the beach.

5 reasons to get a pet

It's estimated that 69 per cent of all Australian households own a pet, and it's easy to see why. Whether it's a dog, cat, bird or fish, pets keep us company, provide a sense of purpose and teach us valuable life lessons. Assistance dogs take it one step further and support people with chronic conditions like epilepsy, vision loss, diabetes and mental illness. Here are some of the health and wellbeing benefits that come with pet ownership.

1 Health perks Pet owners are generally more physically active than those who don't own pets. In particular, dog owners benefit from taking their pets for regular walks or throwing balls for them. Even less active pets like cats, birds and fish need to be fed and cared for, which helps assist with our own mobility.

2 Social benefits Pets create plenty of opportunities for social interactions, whether that's stopping for pats on your daily walks, chatting to fellow pet owners at the vet or serving as a conversation-starter with visitors to your home.

3 Stress reduction When you pat, cuddle or engage with a pet, it releases the feel-good hormone oxytocin in the brain, helping you to feel relaxed and reducing feelings of stress, anxiety and depression.

4 Allergy prevention Research shows that having a furry pet in your home during a child's first year of life can reduce the child's chance of developing hay fever, asthma or eczema later in life. It can also contribute to a stronger immune system and fewer ear infections.

5 Affection and companionship One of the biggest benefits of owning a pet is the company they provide. Many people consider their pets as part of the family, a loyal companion that gives them a sense of purpose. Pets also help reduce feelings of loneliness and isolation.

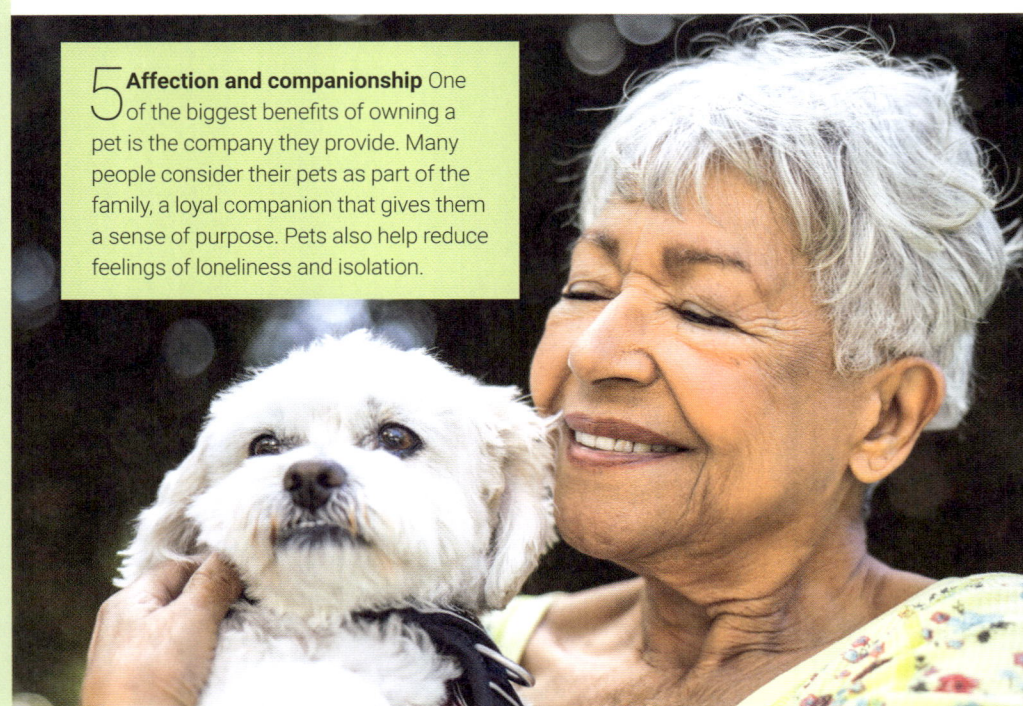

Spotlight on alcohol

ARE YOU DRINKING TOO MUCH?

If you're exceeding the Australian Guidelines (see below) or your drinking is interfering with relationships, work or your health in any way, you may benefit from cutting back.

Ask yourself these questions:

Q Have you noticed a decline in your sleep patterns, lack of energy, increased anxiety or decreased immunity, directly related to your alcohol consumption?
Q Do you view alcohol as a reward or a way to alleviate boredom or loneliness?
Q Do you find yourself thinking about alcohol frequently or planning activities that revolve around drinking?
Q Have you ever experienced blackouts or memory lapses after drinking?
Q Do you wake up with feelings of guilt or remorse after a night of drinking?
Q Does your mood or behaviour change in a concerning way when drinking, such as becoming aggressive, emotional or reckless or losing your inhibitions?
Q Have you ever hidden or minimised your alcohol consumption to others, including healthcare professionals?

If you answered "yes" to any of these questions, it might be time to reassess the role that alcohol plays in your life.

BENEFITS TO CUTTING BACK

Drinking less can lead to better health and wellbeing. Cutting back on alcohol in the short term can improve things like sleep, energy levels, mental wellbeing and memory. And in the long-term, drinking less can reduce the risk of developing:

- several types of cancer including throat, mouth, liver, breast and bowel cancer
- heart disease and stroke
- osteoporosis
- liver disease
- pancreatitis
- gastrointestinal disease.

TIPS TO REDUCE YOUR DRINKING

- Set yourself a drink limit and stick to it.
- Have a few alcohol-free days each week.
- Make every second drink non-alcoholic.
- Keep less alcohol at home.
- Don't let others top up your glass for you.
- Avoid shouting rounds with friends.

TIPS TO TAKE A BREAK FROM ALCOHOL

- Practise ways to say no to drinks.
- Organise alcohol-free events with friends.
- Choose mocktails or non-alcoholic mixers.
- Avoid situations where you might be tempted to drink or plan distractions for the times of day when you drink the most.
- See your doctor for advice or support.

THE GUIDELINES

The National Health and Medical Research Council recommends the following to reduce the risks for healthy adults over the age of 18:
- No more than 10 standard drinks a week
- No more than 4 standard drinks on any one day

Avoid drinking alcohol while planning a pregnancy, during pregnancy and while breastfeeding.

Red or white wine (150ml)	Schooner of beer (425ml)	Stubby of beer (375ml)	Shot of spirits (30ml)	Cocktail (60-90ml)	Champagne (150ml)
STANDARD DRINKS					
11.5 to 13.5% alcohol	4.8% alcohol	3.5% alcohol	40% alcohol	40% alcohol	12% alcohol 150ml =
1.5 drinks	**1.6 drinks**	**1 drink**	**1 drink**	**2-3 drinks**	**1.4 drinks**

For more information, visit the Alcohol and Drug Foundation; adf.org.au

Mindfulness activities for the whole family

Practising mindfulness is a great way to ease stress, combat anxiety and be more present and engaged in what's happening around us. Try these ideas suited to all ages.

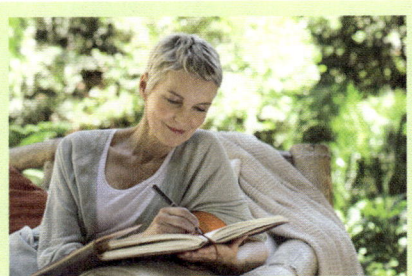

Keep a gratitude journal and add three to five things that you're grateful for each day. You might like to do this first thing in the morning to start your day on a positive note or before bed as a way to process the day and wind down.

Breathe like a dragon. Take a deep breath through the nose, filling your belly and chest, and exhale forcefully through your mouth, just like a fire-breathing dragon.

Do some colouring to focus on the present, disconnect from worries and embrace the imperfect. Tune into the sound and sensation of the pencil crayon on paper, the vibrant colours and the joy of creativity.

Puzzles require focus, attention to detail and presence of mind – all key components of mindfulness. They're also fun and rewarding. Try jigsaw puzzles, crosswords, Wordle, Sudoku, riddles or spot the differences.

Body scanning is a simple form of meditation that can help build self-awareness and calm the mind and body. Lie down and breathe slowly while mentally 'scanning' your body from head to toe, tuning into the different sensations you feel at each point.

Try single-tasking. Choose one urgent task that might be weighing on your mind and put all of your focus into completing it. Minimise distractions and set timers to block out the time required to achieve your task.

Eat mindfully. Fully appreciate your meals by removing all distractions and enjoying your food in silence. Chew slowly and focus on the flavours, textures and aromas of each bite, acknowledging the time and effort that went into the meal's preparation.

Go for a nature walk. Head outside for a walk in the bush, along the beach or around the neighbourhood. Stop along the way to observe plants, rocks, birds or colours, taking note of what you see, hear and feel.

Music appreciation. Choose a song and listen to it in a comfortable space where you won't be interrupted (you may like to wear headphones). Take notice of the lyrics, the different sounds and instruments you hear and the way the music makes you feel.

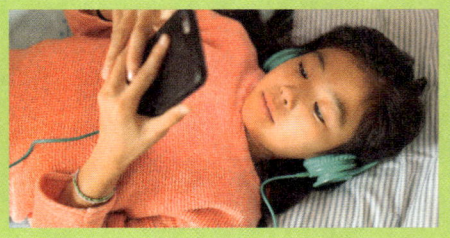

Subscribe to *The Australian Women's Weekly*

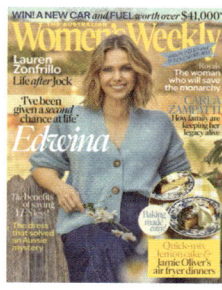 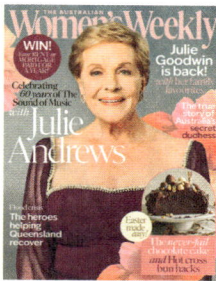 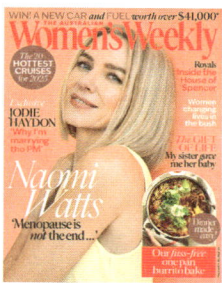

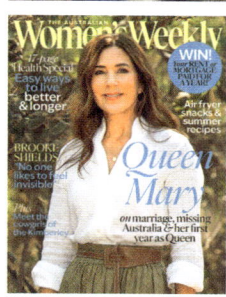 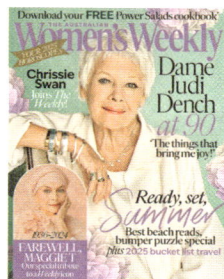 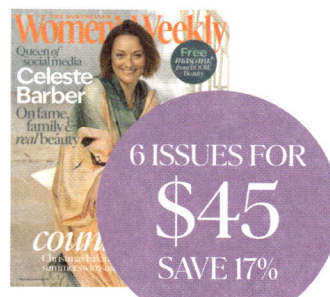

6 ISSUES FOR $45 SAVE 17%

Subscribe & Receive

- 6 ISSUES of *The Australian Women's Weekly* for $45 via automatic renewal
- SAVE 17% off the retail price
- FREE home delivery each month

Subscribe today

magshop.com.au/awwhealth26
or call
136 116 and quote
M253WHD

Savings based on *The Australian Women's Weekly* cover price of $8.99. For full terms and conditions, visit magshop.com.au/AWWHEALTH26. Offer valid from 1st September, 2025 to 31st December, 2026 to Australian residents only 18 years or over. Subscription copies do not receive free gifts offered at retail. Our Privacy Policy can be found at aremedia.com.au/privacy and includes important information about our collection, use and disclosure of your personal information (including the provision of targeted advertising based on your online activities). It explains that if you do not provide us with information we have requested from you, we may not be able to provide you with the goods and services you require. It also explains how you can access or seek correction of your personal information, how you can complain about a breach of the Australian Privacy Principles and how we will deal with a complaint of that nature. If you elect the automatic renewal payment term, your subscription is subject to continued auto-renewal. Your credit card will continue to be charged as per the above rate and term unless you cancel, and is subject to any price increases notified to you in accordance with the Magshop terms and conditions. For full Magshop terms and conditions including auto-renewal payment plan terms, please visit magshop.com.au/terms. Please allow up to 6 weeks to receive your first issue.

	NOVEMBER					
S	M	T	W	T	F	S
1	2	3	4	5	6	7
8	9	10	11	12	13	14
15	16	17	18	19	20	21
22	23	24	25	26	27	28
29	30					

	DECEMBER					
S	M	T	W	T	F	S
		1	2	3	4	5
6	7	8	9	10	11	12
13	14	15	16	17	18	19
20	21	22	23	24	25	26
27	28	29	30	31		

	JANUARY					
S	M	T	W	T	F	S
31					1	2
3	4	5	6	7	8	9
10	11	12	13	14	15	16
17	18	19	20	21	22	23
24	25	26	27	28	29	30

30 MONDAY

1 TUESDAY

2 WEDNESDAY

3 THURSDAY

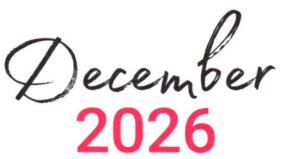
December 2026

4 FRIDAY

5 SATURDAY HANUKKAH BEGINS

BUY YOUR 2027 DIARY TODAY
and help support breast cancer research. Visit breastcancer trials.org.au, and grab a few extra copies as Christmas gifts.

6 SUNDAY

		N	O V	E M	B E	R	
S	M	T	W	T	F	S
1	2	3	4	5	6	7
8	9	10	11	12	13	14
15	16	17	18	19	20	21
22	23	24	25	26	27	28
29	30					

		D E C	E M	B E	R	
S	M	T	W	T	F	S
		1	2	3	4	5
6	7	8	9	10	11	12
13	14	15	16	17	18	19
20	21	22	23	24	25	26
27	28	29	30	31		

		J A N	U A	R Y		
S	M	T	W	T	F	S
31					1	2
3	4	5	6	7	8	9
10	11	12	13	14	15	16
17	18	19	20	21	22	23
24	25	26	27	28	29	30

7 MONDAY

8 TUESDAY

9 WEDNESDAY

10 THURSDAY

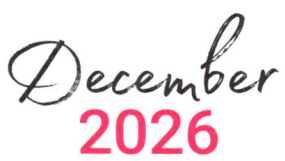
December 2026

11 FRIDAY

12 SATURDAY

AVOID THE MID-AFTERNOON ENERGY SLUMP by eating a lunch that contains protein and carbohydrates. Try a tuna sandwich, homemade lasagne or a lentil and vegetable dhal.

13 SUNDAY

	NOVEMBER					
S	M	T	W	T	F	S
1	2	3	4	5	6	7
8	9	10	11	12	13	14
15	16	17	18	19	20	21
22	23	24	25	26	27	28
29	30					

	DECEMBER					
S	M	T	W	T	F	S
		1	2	3	4	5
6	7	8	9	10	11	12
13	14	15	16	17	18	19
20	21	22	23	24	25	26
27	28	29	30	31		

	JANUARY					
S	M	T	W	T	F	S
31					1	2
3	4	5	6	7	8	9
10	11	12	13	14	15	16
17	18	19	20	21	22	23
24	25	26	27	28	29	30

14 MONDAY

15 TUESDAY

16 WEDNESDAY

17 THURSDAY

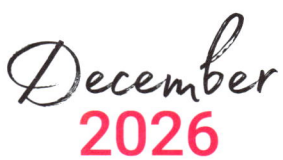

December 2026

18 FRIDAY

19 SATURDAY

WORRIED ABOUT YOUR ALCOHOL INTAKE? Try the Drink Tracker, My Drink Check tool or Daybreak app at hellosunday morning.org to make a positive change.

20 SUNDAY

	NOVEMBER					
S	M	T	W	T	F	S
	1	2	3	4	5	6	7
8	9	10	11	12	13	14
15	16	17	18	19	20	21
22	23	24	25	26	27	28
29	30					

	DECEMBER					
S	M	T	W	T	F	S
		1	2	3	4	5
6	7	8	9	10	11	12
13	14	15	16	17	18	19
20	21	22	23	24	25	26
27	28	29	30	31		

	JANUARY					
S	M	T	W	T	F	S
31					1	2
3	4	5	6	7	8	9
10	11	12	13	14	15	16
17	18	19	20	21	22	23
24	25	26	27	28	29	30

21 MONDAY

22 TUESDAY

23 WEDNESDAY

24 THURSDAY CHRISTMAS EVE

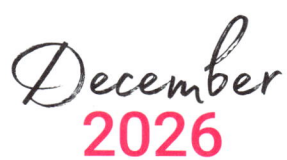

December 2026

25 FRIDAY CHRISTMAS DAY

26 SATURDAY BOXING DAY, PROCLAMATION DAY (SA)

> **CHRISTMAS IS A SPECIAL TIME** to give thanks, to reflect on what we're grateful for and to spend time giving back to others.

27 SUNDAY

		NOVEMBER				
S	M	T	W	T	F	S
1	2	3	4	5	6	7
8	9	10	11	12	13	14
15	16	17	18	19	20	21
22	23	24	25	26	27	28
29	30					

		DECEMBER				
S	M	T	W	T	F	S
		1	2	3	4	5
6	7	8	9	10	11	12
13	14	15	16	17	18	19
20	21	22	23	24	25	26
27	28	29	30	31		

		JANUARY				
S	M	T	W	T	F	S
31					1	2
3	4	5	6	7	8	9
10	11	12	13	14	15	16
17	18	19	20	21	22	23
24	25	26	27	28	29	30

28 MONDAY BOXING DAY/PROCLAMATION DAY HOLIDAY

29 TUESDAY

30 WEDNESDAY

31 THURSDAY NEW YEAR'S EVE

January 2027

1 FRIDAY NEW YEAR'S DAY

2 SATURDAY

> **PREPARE FOR YOUR BEST YEAR YET** by setting small, achievable goals, making more time for self-care and expanding your horizons with a new hobby.

3 SUNDAY

Notes